RELIGIOUS DOCTRINE
AND
MEDICAL PRACTICE

R C
4 8
B3.3
1958

RELIGIOUS DOCTRINE
AND
MEDICAL PRACTICE

By

RICHARD THOMAS BARTON
M.B., B.S., M.D., F.A.C.S.

Associate Consultant
University of California

Foreword by

RAYMOND B. ALLEN, M.D.

Chancellor, University of California
at Los Angeles

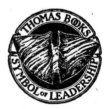

CHARLES C THOMAS · PUBLISHER
Springfield · Illinois · U.S.A.

CHARLES C THOMAS · PUBLISHER

BANNERSTONE HOUSE

301-327 East Lawrence Avenue, Springfield, Illinois, U.S.A.

Published simultaneously in the British Commonwealth of Nations by

BLACKWELL SCIENTIFIC PUBLICATIONS, LTD., OXFORD, ENGLAND

Published simultaneously in Canada by

THE RYERSON PRESS, TORONTO

With THOMAS BOOKS *careful attention is given to all details
of manufacturing and design. It is the Publisher's desire to
present books that are satisfactory as to their physical qualities
and artistic possibilities and appropriate for their particular use.*
THOMAS BOOKS *will be true to those laws of quality that assure
a good name and good will.*

Printed in the United States of America

For

P. C. B.

FOREWORD

By

RAYMOND B. ALLEN, M.D.

The healing arts of medicine and of religion were born in antiquity and their practices were often conjoint. As Dr. Barton points out in this concise volume, institutions of some religions today offer medical services, and even medical education. A man of universal genius, Dr. Albert Schweitzer, practices the art of medicine as a Christian missionary among a primitive people of Africa. With one hand he builds and runs his hospital, brings healing to patients, commits his catholic learning and experience to paper and plays the pipe organ; with the other he organizes the continuing fight against the encroaching jungle.

Our jungles are different. Paradoxically they are not infrequently the by-products of civilization. Besides sickness of body, there is the sickness of mind and soul. The symptoms are anxiety, fear, and hate. The etiology is selfishness. The cure is selflessness. Men of medicine and men of religion should join hands, each applying his skills and human understandings, his God-given insights, to make men whole.

Every man must have something of value in which he deeply believes. When this is a matter of doctrine or dogma of his church, synagogue or mosque no man, certainly not a physician, should intrude upon it. This book is an important contribution to effective teamwork, a practical guide to the physician in accommodating himself to the doctrines and practices of the world's principal religions as he practices his healing arts.

Office of the Chancellor
University of California
Los Angeles

PREFACE

Religion has evolved through the centuries in many directions and has taken myriad forms with a complete lack of uniformity. This book is written, therefore, to serve as a practical guide primarily for the physician but also for the nurse, the dietitian, and the medical administrator, who is confronted by religious beliefs and doctrinal habits with which he is unfamiliar. It is designed to provide a reference for questions of religious dogma as they pertain to the practice of medicine. The main difficulty in this respect is the inability to generalize about categories of religions or about individual faiths, because of the great differences in the beliefs of various sects within a great religion and the discrepancy between the teachings of the founder and the actual practice.

My concern has been primarily with those present-day religious bodies which are sufficiently sizeable to be encountered generally in the United States. According to the most accurate recent census[1] of United States church membership, there were a total of 100,162,529 Americans affiliated with religious bodies in 1955. The following denominational breakdown was also found in the survey—

Buddhists	63,000
Old Catholic and Polish National Catholic	367,370
Jews	5,500,000
Eastern Orthodox	2,386,945
Roman Catholics	33,396,647
Protestants	58,448,567

Let me emphasize that the historical portions of this book are not intended to be complete, but are written simply to help the reader understand the present concepts from their origin, i.e. their genealogy. The text has been compiled impartially as a reference book, not a critique, and the manuscript has been read by leaders of each religious body. I am most grateful for their cooperation. Their viewpoint may, in certain instances, be apologetic, but it

---

[1] *Yearbook of American Churches.* Edited by B. Y. Landis. New York, National Council of Churches of Christ in U.S.A., Office of Publication and Distribution, 1957.

nevertheless represents the present-day rationale of the theology.

The need for such a book has become greater each year in our more cosmopolitan communities and especially in a university community such as mine. For example, the physician or the dietitian may be puzzled by such questions as these when he is ordering a diet for his patients: Does a Jew eat ham? When may not a Catholic eat meat? If Seventh-Day Adventists do not eat meat, do they eat dairy products? Will they take liver injections?

Recently, a man underwent an operation which often-times necessitates a blood transfusion. When I told him this afterwards he retorted, "You wouldn't have given me any blood! I wouldn't let you. I don't believe in transfusions!" This man was a member of Jehovah's Witnesses. Had I known of their belief in this regard, I certainly would have come to some understanding pre-operatively or I never would have contemplated surgery upon him.

These then are some of the situations wherein this book may prove of value. A portion of the material is derived from lectures given at the University of California at Los Angeles and other institutions, but it is herein compiled for the first time as a handbook.

R. T. B.

ACKNOWLEDGMENTS

The author records his appreciation to the following for their criticism of the manuscript in connection with portions of this book:

To *Dr. Bawa P. Singh,* Instructor at the University of California at Los Angeles School of Medicine, and to *Ramu Pandit* of the University of Southern California, Hinduism; to *Hitoshi Tsufura,* Director of the National Young Buddhist Association, *Dean Alan Watts,* formerly of the American Academy of Asian Studies, both of San Francisco, and to *Bhikshu Shinkaku* of the Soto Zen Temple, Honolulu, T. H., Buddhism; to *Rabbi Rudolph Lupo* of the Peter M. Kahn Memorial Jewish Community Library; to *Dr. Mohammed Modjallal,* Professor of Medicine at the University of Teheran, Islam; to the *Reverend A. Homer Demopulos* of Saint Sophia Cathedral in Los Angeles, Eastern Orthodox; to *Horace Holley,* Secretary of the National Spiritual Assembly of the Bahais of the United States in Wilmette, Illinois; to *Darrell F. X. Finnegan, S. J.,* Chairman of the Department of Education at Loyola University of Los Angeles, and to *Rev. Carl Gerkan* of the Cathedral of St. Vibiana, Roman Catholicism; to *Dr. Edgar J. Goodspeed,* Professor Emeritus of Religion at the University of Chicago, *Dr. Henry J. Cadbury* of Haverford College, Haverford, Pennsylvania, and *Rev. Bertrand Hause* of the Religion and Health Research Department of the Hospital of the Good Samaritan of Los Angeles, Christian Protestantism; to *Owen Scranton,* Congregation Servant of Hawthorne, California, Jehovah's Witnesses; to *President Fred S. Williams,* Director of the Bureau of Information at the Los Angeles Temple of the Church of Jesus Christ of Latter-Day Saints; to *Elder G. A. Stevens* of the Glendale Seventh-Day Adventist Church and *Dr. DeWitt Fox,* Editor of *Life and Health* magazine, Washington, D. C.; to *Charles L. Reilly,* of the Committee on Publication for Southern California, Christian Science; to *Dr. Sue Sikking,* Director of Unity-by-the-Sea; and to *Dr. Frederick Mayer* of the

Department of Philosophy at University of Redlands for his help on the Religions of Healthy-Mindedness.

Also, the author herein acknowledges special appreciation for general criticism to *Dr. Floyd Ross* of the School of Religion, University of Southern California, and to *Dr. Raymond B. Allen* of the University of California for his encouragement and inspiration.

R. T. B.

TABLE OF CONTENTS

RELIGIOUS DOCTRINE
AND
MEDICAL PRACTICE

I

HISTORY:
THE RELIGIOUS APPROACH TO HEALING

There is evidence that goes as far back as seven or eight thousand years ago, when man first began to write, that the leaders of the primitive groups of people were the first "specialists." They were priests, doctors, teachers, and policemen all combined. As civilization evolved, these physician-priests presided from an armamentarium of magic and superstition.

The realization that mortal death is inevitable undoubtedly initiated early religion; and when it very soon became obvious to man that certain ailments were related to the mind and behavior, a belief developed that sickness was the consequence of offenses to a variety of gods. The worship, fear, and sacrifices for these deities became an important part of the ancient thinking, and the physician-priest was therefore dedicated to placating these gods.

Thus, religion and medicine were virtually one and the same thing through many centuries of man's history, and some physician-priests were actually deified. "Doctor" Imhotep was probably the first physician in recorded history (3000 B.C.), and was made an Egyptian god in 525 B.C. It is from his influence that the Greek Asclepian cult and the god of healing, Esmun, in the Semitic peoples of Syria, Palestine, and Phoenicia evolved.

Asclepius was one of the highest conceptions of Greek gods. He was pure, above scandal, available to all of ill-health, and his death for the love of mankind was not unlike that of Jesus. The Gerasa Statue of Asclepius became in the fifth century A.D. with the popularization of Christianity the first sculptured representation of the Christ. Thus, because of the benignity and kindness that the ancient Greeks attributed to the physician Asclepius, and portrayed in his statues, his likeness survives in the Christian conception of the savior of mankind.

That a physician named Asclepius actually lived in ancient Greece is likely.[1] However, the mythology deifying him is simply part of the archaic Greek religious fabrications. Nevertheless, the cult of Asclepius was the only one to survive the inroads of Christianity and it was considered Christianity's most dangerous enemy. Christ and Asclepius were much alike in that both had mortal mothers but divine fathers, both were considered healers and saviors of mankind, both lived pure lives, and both died for the love of man. The argument between the two groups of followers was bitter, and the only true reproach which the church fathers could bring against Asclepius was that he was of illegitimate birth. However, the pagans did not mind that much, since they could with equal justification return the compliment.

So it is seen that this body of belief, magic, superstition, and tradition, which was both religion and medicine, persisted for centuries up to about twenty-five hundred years ago. At that time it began to undergo a gradual (over centuries) sort of "binary fission." The dichotomy was apparent by 400 B.C. when Hippocrates first denied the super-natural or sacred origin of disease.

Epilepsy had up to his time been considered "the sacred disease," because it was thought that epileptics were harboring spirits or gods which made them behave strangely. These individuals were often venerated for their seizures. Hippocrates made a pertinent observation saying, "It seems to me that the disease (epilepsy) is no more divine than any other. It has a natural cause just as other diseases have. *Men think it is divine only because they do not understand it.*"

It is at this point in history that religion and scientific medicine parted philosophically. For as Feynman[2] of the California Institute of Technology has pointed out, the reason for this disassociation is that it is imperative for the scientist to doubt and to admit that he does not know. Whereas most religion demands absolute belief. The teaching of Hippocrates demonstrated disease to be a natural process the outcome of which was recovery, chro-

---

[1] Webb, J. C.: The Mythology of Asclepius. Los Angeles, *The University of Southern California Medical Bulletin*, 8:12-22 (Oct.) 1955.

[2] Feynman, R. P.: The Relation of Science and Religion. *Engineering and Science*, XIX:20-23 (June) 1956.

nicity, or death. The priestly contention of primitive times that disease was an absolute, supernatural phenomenon of punishment by the gods for sin or misconduct was undermined.

Today, the scientist works on the theory that truth is "high probability, that it is relative, and that it can best be obtained by the scientific method. Metaphysical conditions introduce unnecessary non-verifiable speculations. The classical philosopher's quest for certainty has led to the scientist's concept of uncertainty, and the study of determinism has brought us to the principle of indeterminancy (Heisenberg).

Metaphysicians speculate about the everlasting structure of things and about the universal criteria of knowledge, but all too often science proves them in error. For example, some theologians have taught that disease has been placed on man because of his sinful past; and that there was no disease prior to this. Others extend the concept to the contention that sickness is man-generated by his evil deeds or thoughts. However, Dawson[1] has shown conclusively that plant and animal disease pre-existed man's arrival on earth by millions of years.

On the other hand, scientific medicine has an infinite road ahead with only a minor portion traveled to date. Its pace has been agonizingly slow with the major progress coming only in the past few years. In the early colonial times of North America, disease was interpreted in Biblical terms and associated with sin.[2] If children were sick or died, it was thought that "original sin" was to blame; whereas if adults were ill or expired, it was thought to be the result of "sinful living." Because of this the clergy played a major role in the early medical practice. Men like Cotton Mather even wrote treatises on medical subjects and the local minister and physician were usually again combined in one person, in what was called "the angelic conjunction."

Two hundred years ago, doctors were conscientiously aggravating their patients with bleeding, purging, and the use of emetics. This, for example, is the unfortunate regime that the physicians of George Washington followed when the First President was dying

---

[1] Dawson, G. G.: *Healing: Pagan and Christian.* London, Macmillan, 1935.

[2] Parrish, H. M.: Contributions of the Clergy to Early American Medicine. *The Journal of the Bowman Gray School of Medicine* of Wake Forest College, Nov., 1956.

of an acute laryngotracheitis. The scientifically-accurate suggestion
of a tracheotomy was proposed by Dr. Elisha Cullen Dick, who was
one of the consultants; but this was rejected by his older colleagues.
Medicine had barely climbed back up to the level of the ancient
Greeks!

Even one hundred years ago, diagnostic techniques were gross
and inaccurate, surgery was crude and unsterile, medicines were
ineffective and untrustworthy, and there was much that was little
more than superstition in medical practice. It was during this
period that most of the anti-medical religious bodies originated.
The improper and inaccurate medical prognoses made many a faith
healer look successful.

Today, medical practitioners still make erroneous diagnoses
and prognoses. In some such instances, the faith healing is credited
with a victory; whereas it is our ignorance as physicians, pretending
to know absolute answers, that proves us wrong. As the *Journal of
the American Medical Association* editorializes (Jan. 28, 1956):

"The medical profession recognizes the power of faith on the
individual mind as a factor that may affect the condition of sick
people. It also recognizes the fact that 'faith healing,' as such, has
no accepted merit whereby it can be regarded as having remedial
or curative effect in persons who are actually victims of organic
disease.

It is true that persons have had what they believe to be relief
or even cure of ailments that must be regarded as self-limited or
imaginary, for the most part. There are even occasional instances
in which diseases generally regarded as uniformly fatal reverse
themselves without any explainable medical phenomena, whether
or not the patient has had the ministrations of 'Scientists' or other
so-called healers. It should be realized, of course, that if such a
phenomenon were to occur to an individual under 'treatment' by
one of these healers, the likelihood is that he or she would take the
credit.

There have been reported in the medical literature evaluations
of 'faith healing,' and the medical attitude is that such healing is
perhaps a part of religious tradition, particularly in the United
States, where there has been a wide variety of religious cults whose
leaders claimed special healing abilities. These reports refer particularly to those individuals, frequently itinerants, who exhort,

pray, and practice 'laying on of hands.' They have also been designated as 'divine healers.' These persons were able to interest others, and may, in cases where no organic disease exists, influence the thinking of many lay individuals to such an extent that they believe they have had curative ministrations.

From a public health standpoint, it is known that such faith healers often display a woeful ignorance of public health measures. Diseased persons mingle in crowds, in tents and other public meeting places and may very easily upset careful scientific efforts to suppress the spread of contagion or infection by accepted public health measures. The further danger exists that persons whose physical condition demands prompt and adequate scientific medical attention may, by delay or abandonment of such care, contribute to their needless early death."

Nevertheless, divine healing is seriously accepted in many areas today. Just recently, the newspapers told of a conflict in the Dutch royal household over the employment of a faith healer in the treatment of partial blindness. At the same time, newspaper and magazine articles here in the United States were exposing the flourishing business of "Faith Healers" with their "healing cloths" and "miracles."[1] Most of these promoters have been highly successful in making money and attempts at convicting them of practicing medicine without a license have generally failed.

In 1954, a commission on divine healing set up by the Archbishops of Canterbury and York asked the British Medical Association whether there was any evidence that improvement or cure of disease, or accelerated recovery from illness, can result from spiritual ministrations. The findings of the B. M. A. committee were that there was "no evidence that any special type of illness is cured solely by spiritual healing that cannot be cured by medical methods not involving such claims."[2] The committee often found that when cures claimed for spiritual healing were investigated the patient was at the same time receiving medical treatment, although this fact was not revealed by those claiming the "cures."

It did acknowledge, however, that the value of religious ministrations in the treatment of various disorders is great. Many of

[1] Kobler, J: The Truth About Faith Healers. *McCalls*, Feb., 1957.

[2] *Divine Healing and Cooperation between Doctors and Clergy.* London, British Medical Association, 1956.

the cures effected by unorthodox means, including faith healing, are mainly due to suggestion, which is more likely to be effective if it has a religious background.

In these cases of alleged spontaneous healing full details of diagnosis were requested, with special emphasis on the nature of the case, i.e., whether organic, with corroborative laboratory tests, mental or psychosomatic. It was considered by the B.M.A. group that many of the case histories would require substantiation before they could be regarded as evidence that anything more than what might be called normal healing had occurred.

The cure of disease is a relative matter, the committee points out. Freedom from symptoms or a remission is often thought to be a "cure" by the layman, whereas the medical standard is restoration of structure and physiology. Disorders of psychological origin may be cured by methods affecting the mind and emotional state and may include spiritual healing, but the committee considered it undesirable and even dangerous to apply spiritual methods of healing without a knowledge of the nature of the disease from which the patient is suffering. *"Most of the 'cures' of organic diseases claimed for spiritual healing may be classed as mistaken diagnosis or prognosis, alleviation or remission, spontaneous cure, or the result of combined spiritual and medical treatment."* As an example, some cases diagnosed as epilepsy are really hysteria.

Physicians often encounter illness that, on the basis of previous experience, should prove fatal, but that appears to resolve unexpectedly without medical treatment. Some cancers have been reported to behave in this way. If such cases were treated by faith healing, they would be considered as "cures." When all these possibilities are considered, it leaves little room for miraculous cures of organic disease by the methods of spiritual healing. "In any event, spontaneous or unexpected cures that cannot be explained are rare,"[1] states the British Commission.

All physicians realize that our methods of diagnosis and testing are not fool-proof and we must keep this in mind when rendering opinions of prognosis. In my own experience, I recall vividly the instance of a thirty-two year old mother of five on whom I performed an emergency tracheotomy. At the time of surgery, she was

[1] Foreign Letters: Faith Healing. *J.A.M.A., 161*:1409 (Aug. 4) 1956.

found to have multiple pedunculated growths in the larynx and sub-glottic trachea. These were removed as completely as possible through a laryngoscope after the tracheotomy.

The pathologist notified me later that I was dealing with a highly malignant reticulum-cell sarcoma. Furthermore, he had shown the slides to two other pathologists who, in general, agreed. They were of the opinion also that the lesion was not radio-sensitive and that radical treatment was indicated to avert a certain early death of this young mother.

Accordingly, I advised the patient and her husband of the grave verdict and obtained a consultation to strengthen the position that a total laryngectomy was the only way out. It was explained that this meant the loss of her "voice box," but that with training she could speak again with esophageal speech.

On the following day, the young woman consulted her parish priest. They prayed at great length for her recovery and the husband arranged for a special mass on her behalf. They both felt that it would be impossible to keep a decent home and raise five children properly without a natural voice. They "went to God for an answer."

On the fifth post-operative day I examined the patient by indirect laryngoscopy and noted that no evidence of tumor was seen but there was still a great deal of edema and hemorrhage from the surgery. The patient told me, however, that they (the priest, her husband and herself) had come to the conclusion to "wait and see." Further surgery was declined. I told her that it was her life and her body and that we would necessarily abide by her decision. The tracheostomy was allowed to close.

The woman lived three years without evidence of neoplastic recurrence. I, therefore, decided to send the original slides to two other cancer centers. Both pathologists stated that this was purely "chronic inflammation," that there was no evidence of malignancy in any of the slides! Today, ten years later, this woman is in optimum health.

She feels that God cured her cancer and I have never told her otherwise. This is a good example of divine healing being credited in an instance of mistaken diagnosis.

Why have I never exposed her "miracle"? Because, beside the still-controversial pathological diagnosis, there remains the belief that some intuitive or "divine" sense led this woman to the proper conclusion in the face of "scientific" opinion to the contrary. This, in itself, might be said to be a "miracle."

On the other hand, the English survey mentioned previously turned up the usual cases in which "patients apparently suffered as a result of delay in consulting a doctor, and, as might have been expected, several of these related to Christian Science teaching and practice.[1] Those members of the clergy, therefore, who hold strong views on "faith healing" make cooperation between the physician and the priest or practitioner difficult.

This London report concludes:

"It seems clear that there are considerable dangers in any suggestion of dual care of the patient. In his best interests he must remain under the single care of his physician, and co-operation with the clergyman is likely to be most beneficial when this is restricted to the practice of the orthodox ministrations of the Church, which can play an important complementary part in the management of many cases. The only exception to this principle is probably in cases of functional disorders in which the physician believes that the priest is likely to be of much greater help to the patient than any physical medicine. Most doctors would probably agree that collaboration between the clergy and the physician is desirable and should be beneficial to the patient. It could, however, have the reverse effect if the difficulties were not appreciated and if either profession sought the credit for the cure. The object is to restore the patient to health, and all means must be used. In physical illness the physicians and surgeons may perhaps humbly be regarded as the instruments of the Divine, and the ministers of the Church must support them in their work and give their patients all the spiritual encouragement possible. It must surely never be a question of prayers before penicillin."

It has been difficult for the scientist to evaluate such things as "the power of faith," the value of prayer, "laying on of the hands," anointing, and divine healing. Sir Francis Galton once made such

---

[1] Lister, John: Divine Healing. *New England J. Med., 255*:435-436 (Aug. 30) 1956.

a study of prayer. By tallying the mean age attained by males of various classes—clergy, lawyers, doctors, tradesmen, etc.—during the latter part of the eighteenth century, he proved that although probably more prayers had been uttered by more people for prolonging the lives of the British rulers (because it is in the Book of Common Prayer of the Church of England), these sovereigns were actually, on the average, the *shortest* lived of all classes. This, Galton contended, proved conclusively that prayer had no efficacy.

It actually proved nothing of the kind, but it does demonstrate some of the variables of the problem involved. A study with a constant set of conditions, proper controls, etc., cannot be arranged to analyze the effect of religious healing accurately, especially when it is the contention that religion is merely an aid to the psychic reaction to disease. Therefore, no scientific evaluation can be made of the miracles of Jesus, Lourdes, Christian Science, yoga, etc. There is evidence that hysteria and hysterically simulated disease is much higher in primitive cultures[1] and undoubtedly many of the Biblical miracles can be explained on this basis.[2]

Certainly, however, prayer may be a very therapeutic experience, whether in public or private, and suggestion of one kind or another has been used since ancient times of superstition and magic. Asclepius and his cult used it dramatically with the technique of incubation and snake-charming. Jesus employed it, as demonstrated by Weatherhead, using spittle and anointing with oil. Emile Coué and Mesmer became famous with their sometimes startling results. Certainly, the modern physician and psychiatrist utilize it. This is part of what Dr. Raymond Allen[3] has called "the God-given insights and skills of the art of medicine." It is, therefore, not the proper role of the physician or psychiatrist to ridicule, influence or alter the religious faith of the patient.

The early followers of Sigmund Freud made this mistake of accepting his scientific observations and his philosophical opinions

---

[1] Trowell, H. C.: Training Medical Practitioners. *The East African Medical Journal*, July, 1956.

[2] Weatherhead, L. D.: *Psychology, Religion and Healing.* Page 41. New York, Abingdon Press, 1955.

[3] Allen, R. B.: *The Enduring Elements in Medical Service.* An Address by Dr. Raymond B. Allen, Chancellor, University of California at Los Angeles, at Alpha Omega Alpha Installation Ceremony, January 3, 1956.

as a single teaching. As a consequence of Freud's anti-religious personal attitude, therefore, many of these analysts were openly opposed to the established religions. Pure science should not be concerned, of course, with religion or philosophy as such. Yet to some extent Adler (a Christian Jew) and more especially Jung (the son of a clergyman) also attempted to reconcile the theory of psychoanalysis with religion. Their ventures beyond the border of the scientific and into speculative philosophy miscarried in much the same manner as those of Freud. As Rabbi Liebman states,

"Psychotherapy is committed to utter neutrality in moral affairs and goes beyond its province when it makes 'value judgments' about the total meaning of life."

The Christian clergy reacted to this attack with a hasty rebuttal based more on ignorance than upon a full analysis of Freudian psychology. Slowly, however, the present state has been reached of "peaceful coexistence," as Dr. R. Finley Gayle, Jr., of the Medical College of Virginia described it at the (April 30) 1956 meeting of The American Psychiatric Association. Psychiatrists generally have learned that religious philosophy is not a part of their scientific domain, and churchmen (especially Christian Protestants) have more and more employed psychiatric information as an aid to pastoral work. However, here Dr. Gayle warned of clergymen "doing therapy," and stated that this is just as alarming as catching psychiatrists in the act of "forgiving sins"!

It is not the nature of this work to debate the veracity of religious cures and dogma. However, most of the religious literature today emphasizes the favorable effect of faith on the psychosomatic diseases. Cures of organic disease are less often claimed. The religious writers stress the peace of mind, tranquility, and equanimity of the religious person, and they often state that a religious faith helps prevent fear, hatred, anxiety, and other such destructive emotions. Truly, religion from a therapeutic view is today frequently considered simply as an ataraxic, and it is on this basis that medicine, psychology, and religion seem to be again joining hands successfully.[1]

[1] Editorial: God and The Physician. *J.A.M.A., 163*:1363 (Apr. 13) 1957.

II

RELIGIONS OF ASIATIC ORIGIN

This group of religions grew out of the ancient traditions of India and represents the same cycle of neoteric religion, reform, and finally counter-reform that we see in most organized religion. Generally speaking, this category of beliefs is basically polytheistic and less systematized than others. There is no centralized authority or legalized act of submission. Rather than being religions of prayer wherein man seeks his salvation through the Absolute Being outside himself (God), these faiths generally emphasize an "Enlightenment," wherein man strives to realize the Absolute within himself.[1]

They often allow suicide without religious condemnation. In fact, in certain instances they even encourage it ceremonially. Furthermore, these theologies have traditionally stood aloof from science and world affairs, but they are undergoing the greatest stress and pressure today due to the new materialism and political ideologies in the countries where they have long been established. The effect on their form of worship and content of their beliefs remains to be seen.

The dangerous difficulties encountered in generalizing about religion are especially seen in this group of Asiatic origin. Their division into sects represents deep divergences, and the difference between their highest teachings and the actual practices of the followers is at times astonishing. In speaking of the virtues of these religions, the modern and exalted concept of the teaching is implied.

HINDUISM

History   Out of the wisdom and spirituality of the people of ancient India during the past four thousand years has grown the religion known today as Hinduism. This, the oldest

---

[1] Hunt, E. S.: *An Outline of Buddhism.* London, Knapp, Drewett and Sons, Ltd. 1955. Page 12.

religion of the world and considered by some[1] as the fountainhead
of all others, is the belief of some three hundred million adherents
in India and an additional twelve million throughout Pakistan,
Ceylon, and Burma. The Vedanta Society in America represents
the western extension of the faith.

Hinduism, as practiced by such leaders as was Gandhi (who is
now being deified), is a system of "God-realization," "self-realiza-
tion" or "achieving union with the ultimate reality" which the
Hindus call Brahman. There is no belief in an "individual soul."
Like most major religions, it has many sects, each following its own
beliefs and rituals, and really represents a league of religions rather
than a single faith. Its philosophy is based on the ancient Vedic
literature.

Brahman is thought to have created each universe out of eter-
nally existing material, not out of nothing as God does according
to Judaeo-Christian tradition. The Hindus take the belief, which
is possibly closer to present scientific thought, that nothing which
really exists is ever destroyed absolutely; things merely change their
form. This concept is considered vaguely like the Law of the
Conservation of Energy in modern physical science by Vedantist
apologists. In addition to Brahman, there is a host of lesser gods,
some of whom are feared and others revered. Examples of these
are Vishnu, the deity of preservation and love, Shiva, the deity of
destruction, and the Ashvins, physicians to the gods. Phallicism is
still a large part of the Hindu rites, as is nudism a custom amongst
the Digambaras Jains.

This religion of Jainism is closely related to Hinduism, and is
a dissenting sect which is extremely influential because its members
are largely of the wealthier class. The group denies Brahman and
follows an intense monastic ritual with even greater emphasis on
non-violence. It was founded as a revolt against the chaos of the
polydemonistic Brahmanical religion of the Fifth Century, B.C. by
Vardhamana (Lord Mahavira) who systematized the faith. He
taught self-reliance and the individuality of the human soul.

Sikhism was also born out of Hinduism and represents a more
militant faith. The Sikhs gained a reputation for ferociousness

---

[1] Potter, C. F.: *The Faiths Men Live By*. New York, Prentice Hall Inc. 1954.

and they have subsequently all adopted the last name of "Singh," meaning "lion." Sikhs are easily recognized as they traditionally wear a beard and a turban. The rather sizeable Sikh colony in central California is from this group. This movement was started by Guru Nanak in the Fifteenth Century as a reformed Hinduism and is often called a cross between Hinduism and Islam. His teachings were monotheistic, and opposed to the Hindu practices of child marriage, infanticide, and suttee (the custom whereby a widow threw herself upon her husband's funeral pyre for cremation with his body in order to demonstrate her devotion to her master).

The Parsis in and around Bombay represent a small residual group of believers in Zoroastrianism, which has numerous coincidences with the Hindu religion, and has contributed much to Judaism, Islam, and Christianity. It was founded by Zoroaster in pre-historic Iran (about 1000 B.C.), but has died out completely in its native country probably because of their refusal to do any missionary work. The doctrines of Zoroaster undoubtedly influenced Jesus of Nazareth in His sayings and teachings, as pointed out by Potter. Their dogma is not pertinent to modern medicine, except indirectly in the disposal of the dead. The bodies are deposited in secluded areas where birds come and devour the flesh. The bones are left to dry and eventually disintegrate. This is because of a doctrine opposing burial or cremation.

Hindu philosophers have been the greatest promoters of syncretism—the idea that the great religions should drop their differences and merge on the basis of common belief. The prominent religious reformer Shri Ramakrishna taught that all religions are true and are simply different paths to the same goal. This Indian passion for a universal tolerance, in contrast to the western concept that only their particular faith is the correct one, appears to be the chief barrier between western and eastern sociologists as well as politicians. The physician must appreciate this Hindu attitude.

Nature of Disease One of the basic beliefs of Brahmanism is that of reincarnation, the concept of a constantly-changing, cyclical world in which individual bits of life, of which man is the highest form, are reborn again and again in a long round of reincarnations. This vital force is thought to pass from vegetables to insects, from insects to animals, from animals to humans, from one body to another, sometimes up the scale and sometimes down, until pure enough to return to Brahman, their spiritual source. It is the belief that suffering and disease is the result of not following the Hindu ethics of controlling desire and turning one's mind on the one enduring reality, God (Brahman).

The caste society, now outlawed but still a part of Hindu thinking, is considered a part of the reincarnation process and one may fall or rise in caste depending on his behaviour in the present incarnation. For example, a Brahmin (the highest level) may drop as low as a pig in his next reincarnation if his misdeeds are sufficiently grave. Also, since moksha, or release from the long series of incarnations, is the goal of every orthodox Hindu, the biggest event in his life is really his death. When an orthodox Hindu thinks he is about to die, he will attempt to go to the holy city of Benares, where, by bathing in the sacred Ganges, he can become free of his sins. Benares, consequently, is a "vast, bustling city of death" teeming with old and sick people. The cremation pyres burn night and day as the corpses are brought to the waterfront to be reduced to ashes. However, love for Benares is true only of orthodox Hindus and does not have much appeal to the younger and educated people.

Role of the Physician   The Hindu in America usually accepts medicine as it is practiced here without religious qualification. However, Taylor[1] has pointed out that in India the approach of the western doctor is considered entirely too materialistic. Their religion permeates all medical care and the technical skill of the physician is considered secondary to his ability to align divine powers on the side of the patient to cure him.

He states,

"The most crucial moment in the doctor-patient relationship comes when the physician completes his examination. Very formally then he is supposed to make a statement of prognosis which enlists divine aid. The equivalent of an incantation is expected, such as 'By the grace of God this patient is going to get well.' The prognosis must be favorable and definite. He can then go on to throw in any qualifications that he thinks necessary."

---

[1] Taylor, C. E.: Country Doctor in India. *The Atlantic Monthly,* June, 1956.

In the Hindu world today, the physician may be of a varied academic background from the few regular medical schools or he may be one of the Vaids practicing Ayurveda, a Hakim practicing Unani, etc. However, because of the poverty and lack of education, quackery flourishes in the Hindu culture. Dr. Maria Selvanaya-gam,[1] recently of the Harvard School of Public Health, states that many people in India still have the idea that sickness is due to the anger of gods. So that when anyone is ill, it is believed that the sick person is being visited by a particular god. She states that the rela-tives often—

"... resort to appeasing that god first and send for the priest, who performs ceremonies and gives a peace offering in the form of coin, grain or coconut. For diseases like plague, cholera and smallpox some people get no treatment for fear of displeasing the respective deity. The result of the peace ceremony is usually awaited for three days. When nothing happens remedies suggested by the old folks at home are tried. After this the village practi-tioner is consulted. He tries measures that are often drastic and crude and may make the patient worse. By now the patient's father or anyone responsible may decide that he should be taken to a hos-pital or a qualified doctor, by which time the case may be hopeless. As an example, a man was taken ill with signs of intestinal obstruc-tion. For the first three days, as usual, religious rites were prac-ticed; home remedies followed, and the village practitioner was sent for. Finally, the family decided to take the patient to a hospital. Unfortunately, that day was the new-moon day, which was not auspicious. The patient was taken to the hospital in collapse eleven days after the symptoms appeared, too late for anything to be done.

In many cases the disease is masked, and the patient suffers from reactions to the crude treatment given him by the local prac-titioner. One day a patient was taken to the hospital with a severe dermatitis and stomatitis. The history revealed that he had been treated by some untrained man with crude arsenic and mercury. Thus, it is difficult to come to a conclusion about the diagnosis.

Some practitioners scarify the painful part of the body with a dirty knife to let out the 'bad blood.' Infection sets in and the patient is eventually seen with a severe cellulitis; when a detailed

---

[1] Selvanayagam, M.: Rural Health Work in India. *New England J. Med., 255*: 25-28 (July 5) 1956.

history is taken, the original disease, such as arthritis of some joint, is revealed.

A boy ten years old was taken to a completely untrained native practitioner for treatment of simple tonsillitis. The sore tonsils were massaged with salt and pepper. Only then was the poor victim admitted to the hospital with a high fever. In addition to these drastic measures most of the unscientific practitioners restrict the diets of their patients, sometimes almost starving them, adding greatly to their suffering and prolonging the illness."

This type of superstitious belief is partly attributable to Hinduism, but, in all fairness, it is found to some degree and form in all the other major religions, past or present. That it is largely a matter of education is apparent from Dr. Selvanayagam's description of obstetrical delivery:

"The room chosen for the confinement is generally the dirtiest and darkest in the house; very often it is near a cattle shed. A confinement is considered a pollution—hence, it takes place away from the cleanest part of the house—the living quarters. Most mothers get help from untrained women at the time of delivery, for there are few trained midwives, not to mention obstetricians, in the villages. Attendants are usually from the barber or other low caste. They do not practice aseptic precautions and sometimes meddle too much and handle the woman roughly; consequently both mothers and babies may suffer from sepsis and from injury. This is one of the main reasons for the high maternal and infant mortality in India."

Therapy   Historically, medical practice in India has been divided between the native system, known as Ayurveda, and the imported Arabic medicine, known as Unani. Although these teachings are obsolete according to modern science, they are still widely followed.[1] They consist largely of an empirical system of drug therapy, but it was from this body of knowledge that modern pharmacology obtained *Rauwolfia serpentina,* the widely used hypotensive and tranquilizing drug.

The Vedas, however, contain "charms" for many disabilities from baldness (Atharva—Veda VI, 22) to sterility (Atharva—Veda

---

[1] Sens, S. C.: Problems of Medical Practice in India. *New England J. Med., 252:* 18-20 (Jan. 6) 1955.

III, 22). Some of these traditions are responsible for the false beliefs such as described in Selvanayagam's article. As for infant care, she says "Weighing the babies is considered inauspicious by some because of the evil-eye theory; if someone exclaims that the baby's weight is increasing, the interpretation may be made that the baby will fall ill and die. The ancient evil-eye superstition is found in the Israelite demoniacal theory of disease too.

The Jain vow to abstain as much as possible from sex acts is another of the rules based on Ahimsa, the doctrine against the taking of life. Jains are taught, according to Potter,[1] "that in every sex act, 900,000 living beings, very minute, of the shape of the human being, and having the five senses, but no mind, are generated and killed."

Diet   As a result of the belief in reincarnation and non-violence to animals as well as humans, the Hindu considers eating beef a sacrilege tantamount to cannibalism. Most devout Hindus, therefore, are vegetarians. However, the Sikhs eat goat meat but not beef and the Parsis have no food laws whatever.

The strict Jain refuses to condone the sacrifice of animals, vivisection, and capital punishment. They will eat nuts, fruits, and vegetables except potatoes, which they believe contain microscopic forms of life. A Jain usually strains every cup of fluid he drinks, to avoid killing a living organism.

Mind Cure   Modern psychiatry is much too recent a development to have an influence on Brahmanism. The ancient athletic and ascetic discipline called yoga represents an attempt by the yogi to withdraw from the world and concentrate single-mindedly on Brahman. This asceticism is a national ideal and its holy men, called sadhus, are highly esteemed. In an attempt to purify their minds and bodies, they are said to have amazing control over the supposedly involuntary functions of the body, such as breathing and the heartbeat. It is claimed that they are able to stop the heartbeat for as long as a minute and hold the breath for hours. This physical control is used as a preliminary to more important disciplines, such as renunciation of desires and control of the mind.

---

[1] Potter, C. F.: *The Faiths Men Live By*. New York, Prentice Hall Inc., 1954.

Supplementary Reading

Bernard, Theos: *Hindu Philosophy.* New York, Philosophical Library, 1947.

Eliot, Chas.: *Hinduism and Buddhism.* London, Arnold, 1921.

Farquhar, J. N.: *The Crown of Hinduism.* London, Oxford Univ. Press, 2nd edition, 1920.

Radhakrishnan, S.: *The Principle Upanishads.* London, George Allen and Unium, 1953.

BUDDHISM

History   About five hundred million people in the world today follow the basic teachings of Siddharta Gautama or "The Buddha" as he was later called when he attained enlightenment. This great agnostic lived from approximately 536 to 483 B.C. Born into an aristocratic Hindu family, he broke from orthodox Hinduism and founded a revolt "to solve the riddle of life."

Buddha carried into his teachings many of the Hindu concepts, such as reincarnation and the doctrine of karma (that virtuous conduct is rewarded in future reincarnations and that bad conduct leads to retribution). His ethical system stressed non-injury, forgiveness of enemies, and friendliness to all. He laid the basis of a moral philosophy (including the "Golden Rule") remarkably similar to the Christian enunciated five centuries later. However, in contrast to the extremes of his religion of birth, he preferred a so-called Middle Way of moderation and calm detachment. This, he taught, may be attained by following the Noble Eightfold Path which consists of: 1) Right understanding; 2) Right intention or purpose; 3) Right speech; 4) Right conduct or action; 5) Right means of livelihood; 6) Right effort; 7) Right mindfulness or thought, and 8) Right meditation or contemplation. To the Buddhist, man is but a bundle of *Khandas,* or elements (physical and mental) constantly changing, held together only by the desire for existence and finally dispersed when the desire is overcome.

The Buddha is not worshipped as a god, but is venerated as the embodiment of a principle of enlightenment, and is considered one of many Buddhas. About two hundred years after his death, a schism divided the Buddhists into a Northern or Mahayana branch, which adopted a less rigorous code of behavior for the common man, and the Southern or Hinayana branch, which held to the orthodox Theravadin tenets. The former group includes the Zen sect which has no theology, neither affirming nor denying the existence of God. Its only liturgy is the act of meditation itself, but this is a vital aspect of every Zen-Buddhist's life.

Although founded in India, Buddhism had virtually disappeared from its native country until a recent renaissance. Buddhism possesses a panoply of gods, and it is interesting to note that in China, of the 72 Buddhas, 29 are gods of healing or of drugs and in Taoism one of the various hells is reserved for the physician. However, these gods are vestiges of old China and considered a contamination by modern western Buddhists.[1] The difficulty with generalizations is again apparent in the instance of Buddhism—do we mean Hinayana, Mahayana, Japanese national Shinto, etc.? The physician today is most likely to be confronted with Zen Buddhism here in America or in the Pacific area and it is this concept and its sects to which we are primarily referring.[2]

Brief mention must be made here for the sake of completeness of the philosophical systems of Confucius and Lao Tzu. These no longer represent a religion but are a code of behavior based on the writings of these two men in the Sixth Century B.C.[3] Confucian philosophy and Taoist mysticism have no direct relevance to modern medical practice outside of China, and we have little way of knowing what the present-day practice is there.

These beliefs are essentially Chinese and, in the **Chinese** culture, Buddhism, Confucianism, and Taoism are harmoniously blended with none of the sharp demarcation into sects or denominations as they are in Western religions. They are all considered roads to the same destination. Confucian society is marked by family and ancestor worship along with nature worship, whereas Taoism is a mixture of magic and philosophy designed to attain harmony with Tao or the "eternal way." This (Tao) is considered the supreme governing force behind the universe and is analogous

---

[1] Hunt, E. S.: *Gleanings From Soto-Zen.* Honolulu, Western Buddhist Publication, 1954.

[2] Suzuki, D. T.: *Mysticism, Christian and Buddhist.* New York, Harper, 1957.

[3] Hutchinson, Paul: *How Mankind Worships. Introduction to the World's Great Religions* by the Editors of *Time.* New York, Simon and Schuster, Inc., 1957.

to the Western concept of God. Confucius emphasized the altru-
istic ideal in somewhat the same manner as the Golden Rule of
Christianity.

Nature of Disease   The Four Noble Truths of Buddhism are:
1) Suffering (ill-faring) is universal;[1] 2) The
cause of suffering is craving or selfish desire; 3) The cure for suffering is the elimination of craving, and 4) The way to eliminate
craving is to follow the Middle Way of the Noble Eight-fold Path.

In the Buddhist concept, disease is called *DUKKHA,* which
means something like "frustration." It is not caused by God or
the Absolute but by *TRISHNA* or a "craving" for the impossible
due to *AVIDYA* or "ignorance" of ourselves. Buddhism sees the
individual as well as the whole world going around in circles help-
lessly in a process called *SAMSARA* or the "Whirl." The cure is
to stop the Whirl by what is known as *NIRVANA.* This means
roughly "giving up the ghost," the ghost being the phantom of
your dead past, and awakening to one's real presence ("re-birth")
through the process of *MARGA* or "the Way" of the Eight-fold
Path. Nirvana then is the ultimate goal of the good Buddhist, and
is an impersonal ultimate reality not like the Christian heaven.
However, there is in some of the Mahayana sects a conception
similar to the Christian hell and a goddess of compassion not unlike
the Catholic Madonna.

Role of the Physician   Buddhists, especially those of the Mahayana branch (Northern) in China, Tibet,
Korea, Japan, and the United States, go along with medical science
and readily apply themselves for treatment of physical disease.
Furthermore, there are no doctrinary rules limiting the type of
treatment, and the eccentricities encountered with the Hindu are
less common in the Western Order Buddhists. As a consequence,
the American physician will seldom have difficulty in following
scientific principles of treatment when dealing with Buddhists
except in those few who still hold to the Far Eastern superstitions
and myths.

---

[1] Bhikshu Shinkaku: *Essentials and Symbols of the Buddhist Faith.* Page 7. The
Soto-Zen Temple, Honolulu, 1955.

Diet   The Buddhist code[1] teaches the abstinence from intoxicants which tend to cloud the mind. Other rules are as follows: "The first rule of diet is to halve the quantity. Most of us eat too much. It must never be forgotten that the actual quantity of chemicals needed daily is very small, and it follows that the purer the form in which they are taken, the less will be the bulk of useless matter to be passed through the digestive system and removed as waste. Reduce your meals, therefore, to two a day, and leave the table feeling you could comfortably eat more. There is much to be said for the occasional fast, or at least, a 'fruit fast,' that is, when nothing is eaten but a little fruit not more than twice a day."

The second rule is to "balance the quality, for too much or too little of any chemical will upset the chemical balance of the blood and in time affect the health . . . The ideal diet avoids all rich and spicy foods or anything preserved or tinned. This is a difficult ideal, but very little thought will enable the average student at least to move towards it."

The third rule of diet is to "avoid drinking at meals. When thirsty, and for no other reason, drink between meals, for drink with food dilutes the gastric juices and hinders the process of digestion. Avoid spirits and wines entirely, for alcohol makes higher meditation impossible. Those drinks in which the amount of alcohol in a single glass is negligible are on a par with smoking, and indulgence in such drugs as are contained in tea and coffee. If you can do without them, do without them; if not, be content for the moment with slowly reducing the amount consumed until the desire for them is dead."

Finally, "remember that diet is essentially individual, for one man's meat is truly another man's poison. Experiment until you find what is best for you, but do not let your habits become too fixed. The perfectly trained body can eat anything at any time or go without. If you should be forced to eat what you do not like or to overeat, do so cheerfully, and the next day eat nothing at all until nature has restored her equilibrium. Provided you do not violate a religious principle, it is far better to accommodate yourself

---

[1] *Concentration and Meditation: A Manual of Mind Development* compiled and published by The Buddhist Lodge, London, 1935, pages 170-175.

to environment than to make yourself a nuisance to your friends and a laughing stock to those who are all too ready to judge a man by inessentials."

Dieting is of major importance with Buddhist monks, particularly those of Southern Buddhism in Burma, Ceylon, and Thailand. They are essentially strict vegetarians, whereas Mahayanas eat meat and fish sometimes. Here again, though, it is difficult to generalize because of the great disparity in the teaching of the various sects.

The modern Zen-Buddhist instructions[1] caution "study your diet but do not become a food neurotic." Their only definite rule is to avoid alcoholic spirits, but vegetarianism is recommended though permitting milk.

Mind Cure   One of the noblest beliefs of Buddhism is a system of meditation and intuition, known as the doctrine of Zen. This is a concept that enlightenment comes, not from the study of the scriptures or metaphysical speculation, but from a sudden flash of intuition which occurs during disciplined meditation. The elaborate rules for meditation are not universally observed, but they represent a sort of self-analysis and self-hypnosis designed to aid the individual in breaking with the past and concentrating upon the immediate. Sickness and failure are thus erased by the preoccupation with the present.

The laymen who practice the meditation of Soto-Zen do so for five to thirty minutes daily during their working hours and it appears to be a worthwhile pause in the day from a physical and psychological viewpoint, beside the spiritual aspect.

In addition to these mental exercises, Buddhists here in America apply themselves readily when necessary to psychiatric treatment. The legitimate sects do not practice healing, although some "illegitimate" ones do.

Supplementary Reading

Buddhist Society of Great Britain and Ireland: *Concentration and Meditation: A Manual of Mind Development.* London, Buddhist Lodge, 1935.
Buddhist Society of Great Britain and Ireland: *What Is Buddhism?*

---

[1] Hunt, E. K. S.: *How to Meditate.* Honolulu, Western Buddhist Order Publication, Third Edition, 1956. Page 19.

An Answer from the Western Point of View. London, Buddhist Society, 1947.

Carpenter, Joseph: *Buddhism and Christianity.* New York, G. H. Doran, 1923.

Chih-i: *Buddhist Practice of Concentration.* Santa Barbara, California, D. Goddard, 1934.

Conze, Edward: *Buddhism: Its Essence and Development.* New York, Philosophical Library, 1951.

Davids, Caroline: *Buddhism: Its Birth and Dispersal.* London, T. Butterworth, Ltd., 1934.

Dawson, George: *Healing: Pagan and Christian.* New York, The Macmillan Company, 1935.

Freed, A., and Luomala, K.: *Buddhism in the United States.* Community Analysis Section, Report No. 9, War Relocation Authority, Washington, May 14, 1944.

Gabb, W. J.: *Beyond the Intellect.* London, Buddhist Society, 1946.

Geikie-Cobb: *Spiritual Healing.* London, G. Bell & Sons, Ltd., 1914.

Goddard, Dwight: *A Buddhist Bible; The Favorite Scriptures of the Zen Sect.* Thetford, Vermont, Goddard, 1932.

Hiltner, Seward: *Religion and Health.* New York, The Macmillan Company, 1943.

Humphreys, C.: *Buddhism.* Middlesex, England, Penguin Books, 1951.

International Index to Periodicals: New York, The H. W. Wilson Company, 1920-1955.

Johnston, Donald: *Religious Aspects of Scientific Healing.* Boston, R. G. Badger, 1920.

Otani, S.: Buddhism in America. *Trans-Pacific,* May 22, 1926, page 4.

Paulsen, Alice: Religious Healing. *J.A.M.A.,* 1926, 1519-1522, 1617-1623, 1692-1697.

Ross, Floyd: *The Meaning of Life in Hinduism and Buddhism.* London, Routledge and K. Paul, 1952.

Senzaki, Nyogen, and McCandless, Ruth Strout, ed., comp.: *Buddhism and Zen.* New York, Philosophical Library, 1953.

Takakusu, J.: *The Essentials of Buddhist Philosophy.* Honolulu, University of Hawaii, 1947.

VanBuskirk, James: *Religion, Healing and Health.* New York, The Macmillan Company, 1952.

Watt, Alan W.: *The Spirit of Zen.* London, Murray, 1936.

Weatherhead, Leslie: *Psychology, Religion and Healing.* London, Hodder and Stoughton, Ltd., 1952.

Weber, J. A.: *Religions and Philosophies in the United States.* Los Angeles, Wetzel Publishing Company, 1931.

III

RELIGIONS OF MIDDLE EASTERN ORIGIN

This group of religions is of Mosaic origin and is, therefore, monotheistic and generally highly systematized, although none have developed the efficient organization found in the Roman Catholic Church. Generally, these religions condemn suicide and refuse religious burial to its participants, but the main concept that sets them apart from most of the Oriental religions and the Classic Greek thought is the belief in one God. "The Lord is One." Christianity and Islam both rest on this concept too, although the Trinity is suspiciously polytheistic to the Muslim. Finally, all of these beliefs are messianic—the Jews still awaiting their Messiah; the Muslims, Mahdi; the Eastern Orthodox Churches, the Second Coming of the Christ; and the Baha'is, the "Messianic Millennium."

Christianity started out as a small sect of Judaism, based on the teachings of Jesus of Nazareth. It was rejected by the Jews, much like the eighteenth century Jewish movement of Hasidism; but instead of vanishing after the death of Jesus, it spread steadily due to the influence of the two martyrs, Peter (a Galilean fisherman) and Paul (a scholarly Pharisaic Jew converted from the Orthodox Mosaic belief).

In the century following Jesus, Greek philosophy had become negative and uninspired, but in the second century the Christian concepts brought in by Paul[1] had introduced a new spirit and power. The character of Christianity began to change from Jewish to Greek and the Christian teaching was greatly modified by this evolution.

Also during the period of the Disciples, the movement was loosely organized about the Jewish synagogue. However, after all the apostles died, a stricter organization developed, so that by the

---

[1] Goodspeed, E. J.: *Paul.* Philadelphia, John C. Winston Co., 1947.

second century a formal priesthood was widely recognized. Later, it was to change again becoming more Roman and legalistic. It is for this reason that we have somewhat arbitrarily placed the Greek Church in the Middle Eastern category and the Roman Catholic in the Western.

Generally, the physician will have no differences with this group, as long as he respects their doctrinal rules of diet and ritual.

JUDAISM

History   The contribution to medical science by Jews has been enormous, completely disproportionate to their numbers. This, no doubt, results to some extent from the exalted position that physicians ("legates of God") have held amongst Jews since ancient times. The Talmud says, "Honor a physician with the honor due unto him for the uses which ye may have of him, for the Lord hath created him . . ." This was not always the case, however. In the Old Testament era, the Jews believed that Jehovah controlled life and health, and that sickness was the result of His disfavor and a punishment. There was the feeling that physical remedies for suffering were a sacrilegious interference with the will of God, that He had caused this condition to teach the individual a moral lesson. However, by the third century A.D. the scientific methods of Greece began to find acceptance amongst the Jews and the belief in demons, magic, sorcery, etc. began to dissolve away.[1]

Later the writings of Hippocrates and Galen, which ruled supreme in the medical world up to the thirteenth century, and the celebrated "Canon" of the Arab physician, Avicenna (980-1037), were translated into Arabic, a language which in Europe was known only to the Jews. They, in turn, retranslated them into Hebrew and Latin, and thus the Jews held the key to medical science of the times. Consequently, at the first modern medical school in Salerno, Jews were found both as teachers and learners. It was this famous institution in Italy which grew into the first European university and was known for its catholic spirit. Here, the Jews were accepted

---

[1] Singer, J. and others, eds.: *The Jewish Encyclopedia.* New York and London, Funk and Wagnalls, 1909. Pp. 409-20.

at a time when they were the object of religious persecution throughout Europe.

Learning from these great scholars, the Jewish teachers and physicians wrote works of their own. They excelled in surgery, medicine, therapeutics, ophthalmology, pharmacology, and toxicology. Maimonides, the great Jewish philosopher, was one of these eminent physicians, and like many others was both a rabbi and a doctor.

In 1422, Pope Martin V exhorted all Christians to treat the Jews with kindness and permitted the latter to practice medicine. Nevertheless, by the end of the fourteenth and the beginning of the fifteenth centuries, Jewish physicians found the greatest difficulty practicing the healing art. It was not until the French Revolution that the status of Jewish physicians changed and they were admitted to citizenship, permitted to study at all western European universities and to practice their profession. The many centuries in which the Jews had been barred from owning land and from many occupations had turned them inward and had developed the skills of the mind.

The origin of Judaism dates back as early as the thirteenth century B.C. and the laws of Moses. It, like virtually all of the other great universal religions, has suffered division into denominational groups of different beliefs. Today, about forty per cent of the United States' six million affiliated Jews belong to Conservative congregations, which stand between the religiously strict Orthodox Jews (four per cent), who insist on the letter of the law, and the Reform Jews (twenty per cent), who have changed the letter liberally.

There is in addition a Negro Jewish sect in New York's Harlem, which follows Orthodox Judaism. It was founded in 1919 by Rabbi Wentworth David Mathew, who taught that the Negroes are actually Hebrews originating in Ethiopia.

Nature of Disease   Judaism recognizes as real all the factors of human personality, and does not negate body or call pain an evil illusion.[1] It does say that the final healer

---

[1] Mendelsohn, S. F.: *Mental Healing in Judaism.* Chicago, Jewish Gift Shop, 1936. Pp. 11, 34-5.

is God. Jeremiah states plainly that disease exists, for if it did not
exist then there would be nothing for God to heal. The Talmud[1]
(recorded between the third and fifth centuries A.D.) indicates
that a disease involves changes in structure and that its immediate
cause is a physical agent. There is emphasis on dietetics and sound
mental and physical habits to guard against disease. Headache is
related to poor sight, exposure, alcoholism, and menstruation.
Eye diseases may be caused by the touch of unclean hands. Heavy
meals may be injurious in a cardiac condition. It is noted that the
eating of unclean fruits or drinking of impure water may introduce
parasites into the body. These are but a few examples in the
Talmud of seeking rational rather than mystical explanations of
disease. Not all of the Talmud is as rational, however. A small
ultraorthodox group still forbids the teaching of Darwin as being
contrary to the scriptures. The Jewish goal has been defined in
the "Sefer Ha-Chinuch" as "a beautiful soul in a healthy body,"
a strongly earth-centered ideology.

Diet   The Kashruth practices are today considered a means of
constantly reminding the people that they are Jews. They
are now followed essentially for "spiritual health." The Talmud
ethics, formulated about 500 A.D., were based largely on the Bible,
and are still closely observed by the Orthodox Jew. Even though
the Reformed Jew usually does not follow the ancient dietary laws
strictly, his tastes by tradition and family training usually are close
to the Kosher concept.[2]

Jews adhere to the Biblical injunction of eating only cloven-
footed and cud-chewing animals, such as cattle, sheep, goats, deer,
etc., and are forbidden such animals as the hare and swine. The
latter had a much higher disease rate in ancient times. Also, only
fish with fins and scales are permitted, and shell-fish (oysters, lob-
sters, crabs, etc.) are forbidden. Here, the ancient rationale was
that finned fish were more able to move about and seek fresh water,
while the shell-fish were relatively immobile and remained at the
bottom in the stagnant water eating refuse. All domestic fowl are

[1] Bernstein, A. and Bernstein, H. C.: Medicine in the Talmud. *California Medicine,* 74:267-268 (April) 1951.

[2] Ellis, Rhoda: *A Dictionary of Dietetics.* New York, Philosophical Library, 1956, pages 70-71.

permitted, if properly slaughtered (they must not be shot). All dairy foods, such as milk, cheese, butter, sour cream, fresh cream, etc. are permitted.

Probably the most important part of the Jewish dietary laws is the preparation of the meat.[1] Tradition has it that blood was forbidden as a food in order to teach the Jew a horror of bloodshed. Therefore, the animal is slaughtered by severing the jugular veins and draining the animal of its blood. Any animal killed by shooting or wounding, or natural death, is considered "terefah" or unclean. The next major step is the removal of the forbidden fat from the hind parts.

After the blood is thoroughly drained from the carcass, the meat is washed many times and soaked entirely submerged in water for half an hour. Finally, it is heavily salted in order to draw off the blood. This does not apply to the preparation of fish. It is a very important part of the ritual that the viscera be closely examined and the meat discarded if any evidence of disease exists.

Rabbis ruled that according to the Bible a Jew cannot eat meat with milk or its derivatives, nor can he cook with milk. He should not take milk or cheese for six hours after partaking of meat. Furthermore, they cannot be cooked or served in the same pot or dish, requiring two sets of dishes. Orthodox Jews will not eat at a table where meat and milk products are served simultaneously. All of these laws were hygienic measures in ancient times to protect against food contamination, and the term "kosher" simply means "fit" or "clean."

As for Fast Days, there is only one generally observed Fast Day, Yom Kippur. On this day the Jew takes nothing by mouth from sundown the night before to sundown the following evening, not even water. During the Passover Holidays there is a special ritual but no fasting. At this time the Jew avoids all leaven bread and legumes.

A salt-poor diet prescribed in cases of hypertension or congestive failure causes difficulties when advised for a person strictly

---

[1] Pool, D. and Chavel, C. B.: *The Jewish Dietary Laws.* New York, The Union of Orthodox Jewish Congregations of America, 1946.

adherent to Jewish dietary laws. Dr. Bruno Kisch[1] has written a recent report of his investigation in cooking the salt out of the meat. Salting, however, is not necessary if the meat is broiled on a fire.

Therapy   The connection of the Jews with the drug-trade of the East in ancient times helped them contribute also to a practical knowledge of pharmacology. The Talmud contains a great deal of folk medicine, but a far greater number of rational remedies. A noteworthy statement is to the effect that a remedy which is good for one man is not necessarily beneficial to another. Special diets, bathing, exercise, fresh air and sunshine, change of environment, avoidance of excitement and worry, and similar rational means of combating disease and regaining health are described in great detail; herbs and potions play only a minor role. The Talmud suggested that a thorough examination was necessary for correct diagnosis. "A physician who treated without examination brought harm."

Moses was probably the first to teach preventive medicine when he laid down rules for the handling of refuse, venereal disease, and the dead on the battlefield. Besides this, the Semitic idea of a weekly day of rest was a great contribution.

Modern Jews are treated medically as are the members of any other ethnic group with the exception of the ritual circumcision. The Shulhan Arukh,[2] which is an orthodox doctrinal source book, describes the following technique of circumcision which takes place on the eighth day of life: 1) the cutting of the foreskin (the chaticha); 2) the moving back of the under membrane (periah), and finally, 3) the sucking of the blood (metziza). The foreskin is cut according to the usual surgical technique, but the retraction of the foreskin is supposed to be done with the thumbnail rather than with instruments. The sucking of the blood has been discontinued and cotton or gauze sponges are used. There is no prohibition against the use of sutures, but the use of the Gomco clamp is forbidden by the Union of American Orthodox Rabbis. Conserva-

---

[1] Kisch, Bruno: Salt-poor Diet and Jewish Dietary Laws. *J.A.M.A.,* *153*:1472 (Dec. 19) 1953.

[2] Pardo, J.: *Abridged Shulhan Arukh.* New York, Hebrew Publishing Co., 1928.

tive Jews use the clamp and the Reformed Jews have no definite ritual.

Unequivocal moral and legal antipathy to abortion[1] originated with the Hebrews, who were exhorted by God "to be fruitful and multiply." Women who practiced abortion were severely punished by Jewish law. This attitude toward abortion was taken over unmodified from Judaism by Christianity. Jewish opinion, like Protestant opinion, is not united or coordinated on the morality of contraception and artificial insemination. Judaism has traditionally frowned on celibacy, regarding marriage and parenthood as "the natural way."

Role of the Physician   The physician has always been an honored and privileged person amongst the Jews, and the ancient saying amongst them was: "A physician who takes nothing is worth nothing." As a result, their physicians received comparatively large fees for their services. Modern Jews still consider medicine as one of the highest callings. The "physician's prayer" ascribed to Maimonides says "May the love of fellowman and the love of my art ensoul me. May not thirst for gain nor craving for fame mingle in my service. For these are enemies of truth and charity . . . Preserve the strength of my body and of my soul, so that I might be unperturbably ready to help the rich and the poor, the good and the bad, the enemy and the friend . . . May my mind be always on the alert. While I stand at the bedside let not alien things intervene to rob me of attentiveness . . . Grant the sick have confidence in me and in my art, and that they heed my advice . . . Banish from their side all quacks and the host of counseling kindred . . . If wiser men wish to teach and correct me, may I follow them and be grateful; for the compass of our art is large and wide. But if zealous fools upbraid me, then let the love of my art keep strong . . . Thou hast chosen me, in Thy grace, to watch over the life and

---

[1] Guttmacher, A. F.: Therapeutic Abortion: The Doctor's Dilemma. *J. Mt. Sinai Hosp.*, *21*:111, 1954.

————————: Factors Affecting Normal Expectancy of Conception. *J.A.M.A.*, *161*:855-860 (June 30) 1956.

death of Thy creatures . . . Be with me in this great work,
so that it may avail . . ."

Mind Cure   A distinguishing characteristic of the Jewish religion is its emphasis upon conduct and character
rather than upon belief, faith, or dogma. This puts the burden
directly upon the individual and probably has led to their great
interest in psychodynamics.[1] From the father of psychiatry, Sigmund Freud, on down to today, Jews have been at the front of the
field of psychiatry. Furthermore, the Jewish layman, lacking the
Catholic confessional and the personal guidance of the Protestant
minister, has turned to the psychiatrist in many instances for help
in his emotional life.[2]

Finally, it is only natural that a group, which has suffered for
centuries as the Jews have, would find the religions of healthy-
mindedness less acceptable. Jewish Science, the theological equivalent of Christian Science, founded by Rabbi Morris Lichtenstein,[3]
has consequently been a rather minor movement amongst Jewry.

Supplementary Reading

Baron, S. W.: *A Social and Religious History of the Jews.* New York,
Columbia University Press, 1952.

Friendenwald, H.: *Jewish Luminaries in Medical History.* Homewood, Baltimore, Johns Hopkins Press, 1945.

————————: *Jews and Medicine.* Homewood, Baltimore, Johns
Hopkins Press, 1944.

Gordon, M. B.: Medicine Among the Ancient Hebrews. *Isis,* December, 1941, pp. 454-85.

Jiggets, J. I.: *Religion, Diet and Health of Jews.* New York, Bloch Publishing Company, 1949.

Landman, I., and others, eds.: *Universal Jewish Encyclopedia.* New
York, The Encyclopedia, 1941.

Marcus, J. R.: *Communal Sick-Care in the German Ghetto.* Cincin-
nati, Hebrew Union College, 1947.

Mason, W. A.: Monotheistic Concept and the Evolution of Medical
Thought. *Phylon,* No. 3, 1951, pp. 255-63.

---

[1] Noveck, Simon: *Judaism and Psychiatry.* New York, Basic Books, 1956.

[2] Braude, M.: *Scriptural Psychiatry.* New York, Froben Press, 1946.

[3] Lichtenstein, M.: *Jewish Science and Health.* New York, Jewish Science Publishing Co., 1955.

EASTERN ORTHODOX

History   The Eastern Orthodox Churches are one of three or four Christian churches which claims its bishops are direct successors of Christ's apostles. In the early Christian Church, there were five Patriarchates, located in Jerusalem, Antioch, Alexandria, Constantinople and Rome. At the time of the separation the first four, which included the larger part of the then Christian world, became the Eastern Church. The formal separation of the Eastern and Western churches is sometimes dated as of July 26, 1054, at which time it came to the point of public excommunications.[1] Actually, it was a case of "who excommunicated whom."

A formal reunion was effected at the Council of Lyons in 1274, which lasted eight years, and another was attempted unsuccessfully from 1439 to 1472. Today the two churches are considerably apart on a theological basis with the Eastern Orthodox containing none of the additional doctrines which came into the Roman Church during the centuries following the separation, such as the concept of purgatory, the infallibility of the Pope, the Immaculate Conception of Mary, and the Treasury of the Merits of the Saints (surplus merits). Government is episcopal like the Church of England. There is a fifth large patriarchate in Moscow at present, along with lesser patriarchates of the Serbs, Rumanians, and Georgians.

Nature of Disease   The Eastern Orthodox concept of sickness is based on the teaching of the "original sin," stating that sickness and suffering resulted from this. However, they believe that God may intercede and alter the progress of death and disease by His divine power.

Diet   Fasting, as a means of self-sacrificing, self-discipline, and will-strengthening is recommended by the Church.[2] The prescribed periods of fast are:

a) Advent, the 40 days before Christmas, when fish alone is permitted but not meat or animal products.

---

[1] Attwater, Donald: Greek Orthodox Church. *Social Justice Review*, Vol. 47, No. 4.

[2] Kokkinakis, Athenagoras T.: *Christian Orthodoxy in the Home*. Portland G O Y A Chapter, 1953. P. 8.

b) Great Lent, the 50 days before Easter when the Orthodox must abstain from fish and meat alike.

c) A few days before the feast of the Apostles, 29-30th of June, when fish is permitted but not meat.

d) The first 14 days of August in commemoration of the Assumption of the Virgin Mary when the Orthodox people abstain from meat and fish.

e) The 29th day of August in commemoration of the martyrdom of St. John the Baptist.

f) The 14th day of September in honor of the exaltation of the Holy Cross.

g) One or more days before one may receive Holy Communion. Six hours before Holy Communion no food or drink, water included, is permitted. Alcoholic beverages during fasting are not permitted except a little wine on Sundays.

However, in case of illness fasting is not kept. Women, during pregnancy and the 40-day period following the birth of the child, are not required to fast. The Eastern Orthodox Churches usually operate on a different calendar and their Holy Days may not coincide with the Western Church.

Role of the Physician   The Eastern Orthodox Churches believe that "Holy Unction" is a sacrament of healing for spiritual and bodily infirmities and is used "while there is yet good hope of recovery . . . not once in a lifetime but often . . . just as we use medical remedies as often as we are sick." The physician does not wait until the patient nears death to call the Priest, as in the Roman Catholic practice.

Bishop Kokkinakis[1] states that "sickness calls for both Priest and Doctor." He says, "The Doctor assisted by Medical Science is trying to cure the body and check its pains. The Priest assisted by the Holy Spirit is giving to the sick the Power of Christ to overcome his pains and resist attacks of disease." "It must be understood, however, that the Priest is never trying to replace the Doctor. He knows that scientific knowledge, in general, and the medical profession, in particular, are not outside the realm of the Providential

---

[1] Kokkinakis, Athenagoras T.: *In the Realm of Redemption.* New York, "Cosmos" Greek-American Printing Co., 1948. P. 104.

love of God. Scientific knowledge is a blessing for humanity."

Therapy   The Eastern Churches agree generally with the principles indicated in the Roman Catholic section. It does not condone abortion; however, when it is the only procedure left to save the life of the mother, it is then tolerated. The Orthodox opposition to contraception is qualified, in that it, too, is tolerated when necessary "for medical reasons." Finally, there is no prohibition against the procurement of the male specimen by masturbation for sterility tests, as the ultimate goal is procreation.

Mind Cure   Divine healing plays a prominent role in the Eastern Orthodox Church with its various shrines for the sick. The most popular of such shrines is the "Panagia of Tenos" situated on the island of Tenos in the Mediterranean, southeast of the Greek mainland. Two other well-known healing centers are "The Parian Virgin of the Hundred Gates" and "Our Lady of Lesbos." All of these are credited with wonderful powers and to their annual festivals come thousands, much like the western pilgrimages to Lourdes. The Church officials used to publish an annual list of the miracles that occurred at these shrines but have now ceased to do so, "as it was considered an advertisement for the Church."

Modern psychotherapy is recognized and accepted as a type of "treatment for our Spirit."

Supplementary Reading

Callinicos, Constantine: *The Greek Orthodox Church.* New York, Longmans, Green and Company, 1918.

Carlson, Martin E.: *A Study of the Eastern Orthodox Church in Gary, Indiana.* A. M. Thesis, University of Chicago, 1942.

Footescue, Adrian: *The Orthodox Eastern Church.* London, Catholic Truth Society, 1916.

French, R. M.: *The Eastern Orthodox Church.* London, Hutchinson University Library, 1951.

Gavin, Frank: *Some Aspects of Greek Orthodox Thought.* Milwaukee, Morehouse Publishing Company, 1923.

Hamilton, Mary: *Greek Saints and Their Festivals.* Edinburgh, Blackwood, 1910.

Harper, Howard V.: *Days and Customs of All Faiths.* New York, Fleet, 1957.

Kemp, P.: *Healing Ritual, Studies in the Technique and Traditions of the Southern Slavs.* London, Faber and Faber, 1935.

Neale, John Mason: *A History of the Holy Eastern Church.* London, Joseph Masters, M.D.

Polish Research Center: *The Orthodox Eastern Church in Poland.* Dilehling, Hassocks and Sussex, The Dilehling Press, 1942.

Sankox, Stefan: *The Eastern Orthodox Church.* London, Student Christian Movement, 1929.

Zernov, Nicolas: *The Church of the Eastern Christians.* London, The Macmillan Company, 1942.

ISLAM

History   The religion of Islam is the youngest of the great
universal faiths and was founded by Abul Qasim
Muhammed Ibn Abd Allah (570-632 A.D.). Muhammed was born
in Mecca, Saudi Arabia, and lived as a shepherd until in his forties.
In 610, he experienced a great revelation from the archangel
Gabriel and was inspired to speak the first sentences of the Koran.
As the visions continued over the next decade, Muhammed became
convinced that he was the prophet of Allah. The number of his
followers grew, but so did his enemies, the Meccan merchants.
These people were outraged by Muhammed's denunciation of the
idols that attracted the pilgrim's trade. He was forced to flee, but
eventually returned victoriously. Within a few years after his death
Islam spread throughout Arabia, across North Africa and into
Spain, across Asia and into the Philippines. Although Islam has
remained outwardly intact, it has suffered schisms like Christianity,
the most prominent of which are the Shi-eh sect in Persia, the
Son-nie sect in the Arab countries, and the Ahmadiyya movement
in India.

Muhammed, however, is not worshipped as a Deity or Saint,
but is revered as a Prophet. In fact, "Muhammedan" and "Muham-
medanism" are terms which are unacceptable to the followers of
Islam,[1] because they leave the impression that they worship

---

[1] El-Zayyat, Mohammed: *Questions to a Moslem.* Washington, D. C., Egyptian Embassy, 1954.

Muhammed in the way Christians worship Christ. "Islam" means "to submit" and "Moslem" or "Muslim" is interpreted as "one who submits" (to God's will).

The Islamic creed is a monotheistic one similar to the Jewish and Christian. It holds that Allah (the God of Islam) inspired His message to different great thinkers throughout the ages, in different lands and different languages—to such people as Moses, Jesus and Muhammed. The Muslims believe that Muhammed was the last messenger of God and His message is registered in their holy book Al-Qur'an (Koran). They deny the divinity of Christ and the trinity, but teach respect for all the prophets before Muhammed. Muhammed himself accepted the Jews as "God's chosen people."

It should be pointed out that the Islamic culture of the Ninth, Tenth and Eleventh centuries advanced medicine to a position of world pre-eminence. Rhazes (greatest of Arabian clinicians), Avicenna (author of *Canon of Medicine*), and Albucasis (greatest surgeon of Islam) are examples of the Arabic leadership. Today, however, there is an enormous amount of magic ("zār") and mysticism in the Muslim practice.[1]

In the Islamic world boys can marry when age fourteen and girls when nine. Polygamy, an old Semitic custom, is legal, recognized and practiced. There is no asceticism. Muslims reject priesthood and do not have an organized "church." They believe in the Last Judgment and at the time of death great care is taken to face the body in the grave towards Mecca and without a coffin, so that the deceased may sit up when the angels appear.

Nature of Disease   Muslims reject the idea of original sin and, therefore, the concept that disease and suffering have resulted from the original sin is contrary to the basic Islamic belief that men are born free. As a practical guide to health, the Koran makes some explicit instructions. For example, the importance of bathing is emphasized and it is included in great detail in the preparation for prayer.

It is also interesting that Muhammed stressed the use of the toothbrush (miswak) and never neglected its use personally. In

---

[1] Tritton, A. S.: *Islam, Belief and Practices.* London, Hutchinson's University Library, 1951. Pp. 149 and 152.

fact, even on his death bed he asked for a toothbrush and expired only a few minutes afterward.

The Islamic belief is, therefore, one that sickness comes from unhygienic living and is not a punishment for sin.

Role of the Physician   The physician is held in esteem not unlike that in the Jewish tradition. However, in those parts of the world where Islam has won many of the simple natives, such as in Africa and India, a great deal of voodoo has entered into their healing practices. The zār dancers are an example of treating illness and insanity by such mysticism. These fanatics are like primitive jungle "medicine men" attempting to drive sickness away by wild dances and superstitious incantations.

Diet   Islamic doctrine[1] demands fasting during the day throughout the month of Ramadan, the ninth month of the Arabic (lunar) calendar. The sick, aged, young children and pregnant women are exempt from the fast.

In addition, during the rest of the year, the prohibited foods are: 1) That which dies of itself; 2) blood, and 3) flesh of swine. The Koran also forbids food over which "any other name than that of Allah has been invoked at the time of slaughtering it." It then goes on to elaborate the technicalities of slaughtering animals, all of which are somewhat similar to the Hebrew teachings. Intoxicating beverages are absolutely forbidden, except in "small medicinal amounts." Only the faith of Islam seems to have been relatively successful in controlling the desire for alcohol.[2]

"It is recommended that hands should be washed before the taking of food and after finishing it (A.D. 26:11). . . . It was the Holy Prophet's practice to cleanse the mouth with water after taking food (Bu. 70:52), so that no particle of food should be left in the mouth. There is also a direction that a man should eat with the right hand (Bu. 70:2). To blow on food or drink is prohibited (Bu. 74:24; Ah. I, 309, 357). Taking of food when in a reclining posture

---

[1] Maulana Muhammad Ali: *The Religion of Islam.* Lahore, Pakistan, Ahmadiyyah Anjuman Isha'at Islam, 1950. Pp. 395-401 and 727-741.

[2] Editorial: Understanding the Alcoholic. *New England Journal of Medicine,* 255:445-446 (Aug. 30) 1956.

is not commended . . . nor eating and drinking while standing. . . ."[1]

Therapy While abortion is considered almost an act of murder, there is nothing in Islam against birth control. Circumcision is imperative as it is with all Semitic people. Otherwise, the educated Muslim accepts modern medicine and psychiatry as "knowledge from Allah." However, a belief is often encountered amongst all classes in the Middle East opposing blood transfusions. This is not a part of Islamic doctrine, but it is a popular myth that the individual is born with just a certain amount of blood and that he never gets any more. Therefore, it is not uncommon for the Muslim to be reluctant to donate blood. This superstition has confronted physicians here in the United States treating students from such areas.

Supplementary Reading

Ameer Ali, Syed: *The Spirit of Islam.* London, Christopher, 1946.
Arnold, Sir Thomas, and Alfred Guillaume: *The Legacy of Islam.* Oxford, Clarendon Press, 1931.
Gibb, H., and J. A. Kramers: *Shorter Encyclopedia of Islam.* Leyden, E. J. Brill, 1953.
Houtsma, M. Th., and others, editors: *The Encyclopedia of Islam.* Leyden, E. J. Brill Ltd., 1929-1938.
Hughes, Thomas P.: *A Dictionary of Islam.* London, Hallen & Company, 1885.
Zwemer, Samuel M.: *The Influence of Animism on Islam.* New York, Macmillan Company, 1920.
—————————: *Studies in Popular Islam.* London, The Sheldon Press, 1939.

BAHA'I FAITH

History This religion has grown from the teachings of its co-founders, Bab and Baha'u'llah, and represents a reformed Islamic movement branching from the Shi-ite sect. It teaches world unity and brotherhood. Mirza 'Ali Muhammad, who afterwards assumed the title of Bab, meaning "Gate," was born in

---

[1] Webb, Mohammed Alexander Russell: *Islam in America.* New York, Oriental Publishing Company, 1893.

Iran in 1819 A.D. As a young man he was a devout Muslim. He was, however, destined to lead a martyred life remarkably similar to that of Jesus Christ, whom he considered a prophet like Moses, Zoroaster, Buddha, Muhammad, and Himself. At the age of twenty-five, he experienced a divine command telling him that he was the Mihdi (Mahdi), whose coming Muhammad had foretold. He was rejected by Orthodox Muslims, much like Christ was rejected by the Jews, and on July 9, 1850, the Bab was killed by a firing squad in the Barrack Square of Tabriz ("a second Calvary"). He was buried in a tomb on the slope of Mount Carmel, not far from the Cave of Elijah. His followers suffered persecutions similar to the early Christians. They were beheaded, hanged, blown from mouths of cannons, burnt or chopped to pieces, yet the movement progressed and grew.[1] Baha'is believe that it was the purpose of the Bab's mission to inaugurate a new religious cycle, preparing the way for Baha'u'llah, its lawgiver and prophet.

Mirza Husayn 'Ali, who afterwards assumed the title of Baha'u'llah, meaning "Glory of God," was born in Teheran on November 12, 1817. He became a convert to Babiism when twenty-seven years old, suffering frightful imprisonments and exile to Baghdad, Constantinople, Adrianople, and to 'Akka. It was in 1853 that Baha'u'llah became conscious of His mission, and in 1863 that *He* announced it to the followers of the Bab, who then were known as Baha'is. His son, 'Abdul-Baha, and great grandson, Shoghi Effendi Rabbani (who died in the 1957 Asian influenza epidemic) have subsequently carried on the leadership of the Faith. Abdul-Baha said, "To be a Baha'i simply means to love all the world; to love humanity and to try to serve it; to work for universal peace and universal brotherhood."

Nature of Disease   The Baha'i teachings are that disease arises from two causes—psychic disturbance and natural causes. Therefore, the Baha'i Faith recognizes psychic treatment for inner disturbances and scientific medicine for other

---

[1] Mead, F. S.: *Handbook of Denominations in the United States.* New York, Abingdon Press, 1951. Pp. 25-26.

diseases. The Scottish physician, Dr. J. E. Esselmont,[1] has written an authoritative study of the Faith. He states that according to Baha'i teachings, the human body serves a temporary purpose in the development of the soul, and when that purpose has been served, is laid aside; just as the egg-shell serves a temporary purpose in the development of the chick, and, when that purpose has been served, is broken and discarded.

Does sin cause disease? The Baha'i answer is, "In the sense of disobedience to spiritual and cosmic law, sin is undoubtedly the ultimate cause of disease, but the 'sin' does not apply to the individual sufferer."

Diet   There are no special dietary restrictions in the Baha'i Faith, although Abdul-Baha stated, "The food of the future will be fruit and grains. The time will come when meat will no longer be eaten." The use of intoxicants, except as remedies in case of illness, is strictly forbidden by Baha'u'llah. Generally speaking, the Baha'i teaching regarding all enjoyments is based on moderation, not asceticism.

Role of the Physician   Baha'is are expected to consult physicians when necessary and follow their advice. They consider Baha'u'llah as the Great Physician, the Healer of the world's sicknesses and pray to Him as a Mediator to God.

Therapy   Baha'u'llah wrote to a physician, "Do not neglect medical treatment when it is necessary, but leave it off when health is restored. Treat disease through diet, by preference, refraining from the use of drugs; and if you find what is required in a single herb, do not resort to a compounded medicament." "There are two ways of healing sickness—material means and spiritual means. They are not incompatible, and you should accept the physical remedies as coming from the mercy and favor of God."

There are no special taboos. They obey all the governmental health regulations.

Mind Cure   Baha'is believe that there are also many methods of healing without material means. "Much more powerful effects result from the patient's own mental states," and

---

[1] Esselmont, J. E.: *Baha'u'llah and the New Era.* Wilmette, Baha'i Publishing Committee, 1950.

"suggestion" may play an important part in determining these states. They believe that divine healing can occur, "if healing is best for the patient." Esselmont contends that both Baha'u'llah and Abdul-Baha were gifted with the power of divine healing, much like Christ and His apostles. He feels that the power of spiritual healing is doubtless common to all mankind in greater or less degree, but, just as some men are endowed with exceptional talent for mathematics or music, so others appear to be endowed with exceptional aptitude for healing. These are the people who ought to make the healing art their life work, he says.

IV

RELIGIONS OF WESTERN ORIGIN

When the New Testament was gathered in its generally agreed-on form in 397 A.D. at the Third Council of Carthage, Jesus was called the "Christ" or the "Anointed One," which was a designation equivalent to the Hebrew "Messiah." Christianity had evolved from Jewish to Greek to Roman by this time, and the tendency to dispute on theological issues was already a symptom of its seemingly endless fission. Even Paul had contested Jesus' own brother, James, who was the recognized leader of the Jerusalem church, on the question of whether Greek converts were subject to Jewish law. Nevertheless, in spite of all the doctrinal controversies, it remained essential to the orthodox Christian denominations to believe that Jesus rose from the dead, and that He was of the same substance as God.

Christianity and medicine had an early association in the Greek physician, Luke, who was one of the two first European converts and accompanied Paul on his evangelistic tours. Although the Christian church has had its conflicts with science since then and still has to some extent at present, it is today a fact that science and medicine have prospered in the predominantly Christian countries. Undoubtedly, the teachings of Jesus have inspired a charity and altruism which encouraged medicine and nursing. Christianity is unique in its tremendous dedication to the care of the sick, providing countless hospitals, medical schools, and clinics sponsored by the various denominations throughout the world.

The demonology and superstition of early Christianity has slowly disappeared through the centuries,[1] and the references of the Bible and St. Augustine to demons and witchcraft are given a modern interpretation as being simply symbolic. Also, the belief

---

[1] Russell, Bertrand: *Religion and Science.* New York, Henry Holt and Co., 1935.

45

in miracles is not as widespread as it used to be.[1]   Feynman[2] has
shown that where the Christian Church retreated, such as in the
conflict with science about whether the earth was the center of the
universe (Galileo), the basic Christian ethics of action on love, the
brotherhood of all men, and the value of the individual remained
unchanged.

Nevertheless, churchmen have not been above exploiting
natural phenomena to their own needs.[3]   For example, they taught
that the pestilence of the Black Death had been ordained as a
punishment for man's sins and this belief persisted as late as 1720
when the last great epidemic occurred at Marseilles.   The Spanish
clergy attributed it to the Opera, whereas, the English bishops were
in favor of its being punishment for the Theatre.   There were a few
clerics who firmly believed that the long pointed shoes which had
come into fashion just prior to the outbreak of the Black Death had
proved particularly irritating to the Divine Maker, and that He
had promptly responded by sending the plague.[4]

Another abandoned sanction of the ancient church was the
castrati.   This custom of creating eunuchs was a common one in
the middle east prior to the appearance of Islam and Christianity.
The Old Testament abounds in references to this; and later, Jesus
said that some are born eunuchs, some are compelled to be, and
"some have made themselves eunuchs for the kingdom of heaven's
sake."   The production of male sopranos was probably introduced
to Rome by the Moslem harem guards.   Pope Clement VII was the
first to use them in the choirs, contrary to the present-day dogma
against interference with the reproductive apparatus.   The practice
was eventually condemned by Pope Benedict XIX in the eighteenth
century, yet some such sopranos were heard in the Vatican choirs
as late as 1920 and perhaps even now.[5]

---

[1] Aradt, Zsolt: *The Book of Miracles.*   New York, Farrar, Straus, and Cudahy,
1956.

[2] Feynman, R. P.: The Relation of Science and Religion. *Engineering and Science, XX:*20-23 (June) 1956.

[3] Shrewsberry, Prof. J. F. D.: The Saints and Epidemic Disease. *The Birming-
ham Medical Review,* No. 7-8, Winter, 1956.

[4] Walker, K.: *The Story of Medicine.*   New York, Oxford University Press, 1955.

[5] Freud, Esti D.: Voice Physiology and The Emergence of New Vocal Styles.
*Arch. Otolaryng., 62:*50-58 (July) 1955.

Except for a few fundamentalists, the battle over another Church-Science issue, Darwinism, is over and the physician-biologist need no longer bother about the Church criticism. Indifferentism and what has been called Modernism or the effort to make church dogma conform to the conclusions of science is seen throughout Christianity today. This has gone to the point that the famous Jesuit priest and scientist, Pierre Teilhard de Chardin, elaborated a theory[1] based on the certainty of evolution and contending that with the appearance of man, evolution has begun to converge toward God. His book, withheld until his death and published without the Imprimatur, contends that evolution is a development of consciousness, ascending towards a Supreme Consciousness in which all individual consciousnesses will someday meet. Teilhard gave the name of "Omega" to this summit!

In 1947, Bedouin shepherds stumbled upon a mass of ancient Jewish manuscripts in a cave near Qumran on the Dead Sea. The scrolls apparently originated in a monastery of a little-known Jewish sect of the time of Jesus, the Essenes. The scrolls have been a great help to biblical scholars,[2] and have emphasized the spiritual legacy of ancient Judaism to Christianity. Some scholars have shown a marked similarity between the Essenes and the early Christians. This former group had a sacred meal, practiced community property, and believed in purification through water.[3]

Finally, here again we see the cycle of the neoteric religion (Roman), reform (Protestant), and thereafter counter-reform. With this reform and counter-reform has also come a closer collaboration with medicine and psychiatry, as exemplified in the recent formation of the Academy of Religion and Mental Health. This new-born association serves as a common point of contact between clergymen of all faiths and psychiatrists, physicians, psychologists, psychoanalysts, and sociologists. Christianity and science have become mutually tolerant.[4]

---

[1] Teilhard, P.: *The Phenomenon of Man.* Paris, Editions du Seuil, 1955.

[2] Rowley, H. H.: *The Zadokite Fragments and the Dead Sea Scrolls.* London, Macmillan, 1953.

[3] Yadin, Y.: *The Message of the Scrolls.* New York, Simon and Schuster, 1957.

[4] Editorial: Near Life, Near Death, Near God. *J.A.M.A., 163*:1358-1361 (Apr. 13) 1957.

ROMAN CATHOLICISM

History   The Roman Catholic Church is the descendant institution from Peter, who was appointed to head His
ministry by Jesus. Peter was martyred in Rome and buried there.
The Bishops of Rome who succeeded him, several centuries later,
became known as the "Vicar of Jesus Christ and successor to the
Prince of Apostles" (Pope). Their government of the Church has
been hierarchal and completely authoritarian; no layman may have
any voice in its government.

Of all the religious bodies, the Roman Catholic Church has
the most comprehensive and detailed code of medical morality.
This is based on the "teaching authority" of the Pope, who is now
spiritual ruler of 470,000,000 Catholics in all parts of the world.
The code for the Catholic Hospital Association is outlined by
Reverend Gerald Kelly[1] in five booklets, and represents the appli-
cation of the moral law by the theologian to the "facts" presented
to him by the physicians. It is the position of the Catholic Church
that if it is proven that these original "facts" were not true, the
moral theologian will revise the answer. This does not represent
a change in moral law, only a change in the facts presented. The
physician makes the judgment, the priest's role is merely to state
the laws on which he must base his judgment, according to Catholic dogma.

The Catholic Church sponsors the most elaborate system of
hospitals, medical schools, clinics, medical missions, etc. of all the
churches in the world. There are in America associations of Catholic hospitals, Catholic physicians, Catholic nursing orders, etc.,
wherein the individuals are indoctrinated with church principles.

Nature of Disease   The Catholic viewpoint is that man is subject to disease and death because the "gift
of immortality," which was given to Adam upon his creation, was
lost as part of the punishment for Adam's disobedience to God's
command. "Illnesses are trials sent or allowed by God but not

---

[1] Kelly, G.: *Medico-Moral Problems.* St. Louis, The Catholic Hospital Association, Ninth Printing, March, 1956.

necessarily punishment."[1] As all men are descendants of Adam, they have suffered the consequences of being born without this special gift. Since, however, both disease and death are natural to man, like other natural causes they can be and are suspended by God at times for a good reason. Such manifestations are called miracles,[2] being "occurrences outside the cause of nature, perceptible to the senses, and explicable only as the direct act of God himself."

Diet The regulations in the United States for fasting and abstinence are outlined in detail in the following two paragraphs.

Days of Fast[3] are required of all over age twenty-one and under fifty-nine unless exempt or dispensed. On these days the Catholic is expected to eat only one full meal with meat. Two other meatless meals may be taken according to one's needs, but together they should not equal another full meal. Eating between meals is not permitted, but liquids (including milk and fruit juices) are allowed. The particular Days of Fast are usually listed in the Catholic calendars and include the week days of Lent, Ember days, and certain other religious days (Vigils of Pentecost, Assumption, etc.).

Days of Abstinence (from meat) are required of all over age seven, and may be complete (such as most Fridays, Ash Wednesday, Holy Saturday, etc.) or partial (such as Ember Wednesdays and Saturdays, etc.). On days of Partial Abstinence, meat, soup, and gravy may be taken only once a day at the principal meal, whereas on days of Complete Abstinence, no meat, soup or gravy may be taken at all.

For the physician, the important exceptions are in those instances of sickness or pregnancy. Catholics may dispense with these requirements with the priest's permission in an instance of grave inconvenience, such as illness, and they need not be confined to bed, house, or hospital to do so.[4]

---

[1] O'Brien, Patrick: *Moral Problems in Hospital Practice.* St. Louis, B. Herder Book Co., 1956, Page 111.

[2] Darrow, F.: *Miracles.* New York, Bobbs-Merrill, 1926.

[3] *The Tidings.* Page 4, March 1, 1957. Los Angeles, Archdiocese of Los Angeles.

[4] *The Tidings.* Pp. 1-3, March 29, 1957. Weekly newspaper for The Archdiocese of Los Angeles.

Therapy   The Code of Ethical and Religious Directives for the
Catholic Hospital Association[1] very clearly points out
prohibitions and limitations upon physicians, nurses, hospital
authorities, and the patients themselves, regardless of religion, who
are in, or working in, a Catholic hospital. The *general directives*
listed are as follows:

(1)   All surgical procedures require the consent, at least reasonably presumed, of the patient or his guardians.

(2)   Everyone has the right and the duty to prepare for the
solemn moment of death. Unless it is clear, therefore, that a dying
patient is already well-prepared for death, as regards both the
temporal and spiritual affairs, *it is the physician's duty to inform,
or to have some responsible person inform him of his critical
condition.*

(3)   Adequate consultation is required, not only when there
is doubt concerning the morality of some procedure but also with
regard to all procedures involving serious consequences, even
though such procedures are listed in the code of hospital directives
as permissible.

(4)   The physician is required to state definitely to the super-
visor of the department concerned the nature of the operation he
intends to perform or of the treatment he intends to give in the
hospital.

(5)   All structures or parts of the organs removed from
patients must be sent at once and in their entirety to the pathologist
for his examination and report. If the physician requests it, the
specimens will be returned to him after examination.

(Note: In the event of an operation for the removal of a
diseased organ containing a living fetus, the fetus should be
extracted and baptized before the excised organ is sent to the
pathologist.)

(6)   The obligation of professional secrecy must be carefully
fulfilled not only as regards the information on the patients' charts
and records but also as regards confidential matters learned in the
exercise of professional duties. Moreover, the charts and records

---

[1] Published under the Imprimatur of Archbishop Joseph Ritter of St. Louis, 1955.

must be duly safeguarded against inspection by those who have no right to see them.

The *specific directives* are important and many. They are based on the principles that direct killing of any innocent person, even at his own request, is always morally wrong, as is risking life, indirect taking of life, and suicide. Furthermore, every unborn child is considered as a human person with all the rights of a human person from the moment of conception.[1] The particular applications are as follows:

(1) *Abortion:* a) Direct abortion is a direct killing of an unborn child, and is never permitted, even when the ultimate purpose is to save the life of the mother. b) Operations, treatments, and medications during pregnancy which have for their immediate purpose the cure of a proportionately serious pathological condition of the mother are permitted, even though they indirectly cause an abortion, when they cannot safely be postponed until the fetus is viable. c) Regarding the treatment of hemorrhage during pregnancy before the fetus is viable, no procedure which is primarily designed to empty the uterus is permissible unless the physician is reasonably sure that the fetus is already dead or already detached.

(2) *Caesarean Section* for the removal of a viable fetus: a) is permitted, even with some risk to the life of the mother, when necessary for successful delivery; b) is likewise permitted, even with some risk for the child, when necessary for the safety of the mother.

(3) *Cranial operations* for the destruction of fetal life are forbidden. Operations designed to increase the infant's chance to live (e.g., aspiration for hydrocephalus) are permitted even before delivery when such operations are required for successful delivery.

(4) *Ectopic Pregnancy:* a) Any direct attack on the life of the fetus is morally wrong. b) The affected part of an ovary or Fallopian tube may be removed, even though the life of the fetus is thus indirectly terminated, providing the operation cannot be postponed without notably increasing the danger to the mother.

---

[1] The Reverend Edwin F. Healy (*Medical Ethics,* Loyola Univ. Press, 1956, Page 93) states that "In 1852 the Academy of Medicine of Paris declared that therapeutic abortions were licit in desperate cases. The decision marked the beginning of the practice of therapeutic abortion."

(5) *Euthanasia* in all its forms is forbidden: a) The failure to supply the ordinary means of preserving life is equivalent to euthanasia.[1] b) It is not euthanasia to give a dying person sedatives merely for the alleviation of pain, even to the extent of depriving the patient of the use of sense and reason, when this extreme measure is judged necessary. Such sedatives should not be given before the patient is properly prepared for death (in the case of a Catholic, this means the reception of the Last Sacraments) nor should they be given to patients who are able and willing to endure their sufferings for spiritual motives.

(6) *Hysterectomy,* in the presence of pregnancy and even before viability, is permitted when directed to the removal of maternal pathology which is distinct from the pregnancy and which is of such a serious nature that the operation cannot be safely postponed until the fetus is viable.

(7) *Post-mortem examinations* must not be begun until real death is morally certain.[2]

(8) *Premature Delivery:* For a very serious reason labor may be induced immediately after the fetus is viable. In a properly equipped hospital the fetus may sometimes be considered viable after 26 weeks (6 calendar months); otherwise, 28 weeks are required.

(9) *Pregnancy Tests:* In all cases in which the presence of pregnancy would render some procedure illicit, the physician must make use of such tests and consultation as may seem necessary.

(10) Radiation therapy of the mother's reproductive organs is not permitted during pregnancy unless its use at this time is an indispensable means of saving the mother's life by suppressing a threatening pathological condition, and not by attacking the fetus.

The directives involving the reproductive organs and functions are based on the principles that the unnatural use of the sex

---

[1] Recently, however, Pius XII said that "a doctor may legitimately halt artificial respiration for a dying patient in some cases, if the patient's family requests it." The Pope defined these cases as when the family might feel that the "attempt at reanimation constitutes for the family a burden which in conscience they cannot accept."

[2] As far back as 1706, Pope Clement XI urged the carrying out of autopsies and the contemporary Msgr. A. C. Dalton has stated that opponents of autopsies and vivisection are heretics.

faculty, such as masturbation, is never permitted; that continence, either periodic or continuous, is the only form of birth control not in itself morally objectionable; and that procedures that induce sterility are permitted only when they are directed to the cure of a serious pathological condition for which a simpler remedy is not reasonably available and where the sterility itself is an unintended and unavoidable effect. The following rules are pertinent here:

(1) *Artificial insemination* of a woman with semen of a man who is not her husband is morally objectionable.[1] Likewise immoral is insemination even with the husband's semen, when the semen is obtained by means of masturbation or unnatural intercourse. Recently Pope Pius XII stated that "artificial insemination is an intrinsic evil which goes beyond the limits of the right which married couples have acquired by the matrimonial contract. That right being the right to exercise fully their natural sexual capacity in the natural accomplishment of the matrimonial (sex) act. The contract in question does not confer on them the right to artificial fertilization because such a right is in no way expressed in the right to the natural conjugal act."

(2) *Castration,* surgical or otherwise, is permitted when required for the removal or diminution of a serious pathological condition, even in other organs. Hence:
a) oophorectomy or irradiation of the ovaries may be allowed in treating carcinoma of the breast and metastasis therefrom;
b) orchidectomy is permitted in the treatment of carcinoma of the prostate.

In all cases, the procedure least harmful to the reproductive organs should be used, if equally effective with other procedures.

(3) *Contraception:* All operations, treatments, and devices designed to render conception impossible are morally objectionable. Advising, explaining, or otherwise fostering contraceptive practices is immoral. Continence is not contraception. A Catholic physician is entitled to advise and explain the practice of periodic continence to those who have need of such knowledge.

---

[1] The Archbishop of Canterbury has recently taken a similar stand, speaking for the Anglican Communion.

(4) *Hysterectomy,* in the absence of pregnancy: a) Hysterectomy is permitted when it is sincerely judged to be the only effective remedy for prolapse of the uterus, or when it is a necessary means of removing some other serious pathology. b) Hysterectomy is not permitted as a routine procedure after any definite number of Caesarean sections. In these cases the pathology of each patient must be considered individually; and care must be made that hysterectomy is not performed as a merely contraceptive measure. c) Even after the child-bearing function has ceased, hysterectomy is still a mutilation, and it must not be performed unless sound medical reasons call for it.

(5) *Sterility Tests* involving the procurement of the male specimen by masturbation or unnatural intercourse are morally objectionable.

The morality of certain surgical procedures is dependent upon the principle that any procedure which is harmful to the patient is morally justified only insofar as it is designed to produce a proportionate good. Usually this "proportionate good" which justifies a directly mutilating procedure must be the welfare of the patient himself. However, such things as blood transfusions and skin grafts are permitted for the good of others. Other procedures covered are:

(1) *Appendectomy:* The removal of an apparently healthy appendix while the abdomen is open for some other reason may be allowed at the discretion of the physician.

(2) *Lobotomy* is morally justifiable as a last resort in attempting to cure those who suffer from serious mental illness. It is not allowed when less extreme measures are reasonably available or in cases in which the probability of harm outweighs the probability of benefit.

(3) *Narcotherapy:* The use of narcosis (or hypnosis) for the cure of mental illness is permissible with the consent at least reasonably presumed of the patient, provided due precautions are taken to protect the patient and the hospital from harmful effects, and provided the patient's right to secrecy is duly safeguarded.

(4) *Uterine Malpositions:* Operations devised to correct uterine malpositions (e.g., ligmentary suspensions) without inter-

Religions of Western Origin   55

fering with the normal physiology of the uterus or rendering the patient sterile are permitted.

(5) *Experimentation* on patients without due consent and not for the benefit of the patients themselves is morally objectionable. Even when experimentation is for the genuine good of the patient, the physician must have the consent, at least reasonably presumed, of the patient or his legitimate guardian.

(6) *Ghost surgery*, which implies the calculated deception of the patient as to the identity of the operating surgeon, is morally objectionable.

(7) There is no objection on principle and in general to *psychoanalysis* or any other form of psychotherapy. The psychiatrists and psychotherapists, however, must observe the cautions dictated by sound morality, such as: avoiding the error of pansexualism; never counseling even material sin; respecting secrets that the patient is not permitted to reveal; avoiding the disproportionate risk of moral dangers.

(8) *Shock-therapy* is permitted when medically indicated.

(9) *Unnecessary procedures*, whether diagnostic or therapeutic, are morally objectionable. A procedure is unnecessary when no proportionate reason requires it for the welfare of the patient; a *fortiori* unnecessary is any procedure that is contraindicated by sound medical standards. This directive applies especially, but not exclusively, to unnecessary surgery.

It is the Catholic attitude that sexual intercourse is the great sacramental act of union and personal surrender of married life and is primarily one of procreation rather than self-gratification.[1] The creative function of intercourse is emphasized in their teachings. Therefore, any procedure or device which alters the natural technique of intercourse is considered immoral. Also, such practices as contraception, artificial insemination by donors, sterilization, "the exclusive use of the 'safe period' without good reason," and all sexual aberrations are believed morally evil.[2]

Father T. J. O'Donnell, S. J., states, furthermore, that, "Although not a few doctors have compromised their profession

[1] Jenkins, D. T.: *The Doctor's Profession.* London, SCM Press, 1949.
[2] O'Donnell, T. J.: *Morals in Medicine.* Westminister, Newman Press, 1956.

by associating themselves with programs of eugenic sterilization
. . . the practice is so clearly unscientific and so obviously
immoral as to scarcely merit mention . . ." The author's
conclusions from the study of eugenic sterilization of the otoscle-
rotic deaf have been reported elsewhere, and the Catholic viewpoint is therein reviewed.[1]

*Some of the special rules regarding baptism, disposal of ampu-
tated members, burial of the dead, etc.* are:

(1)   Except in cases of emergency (i.e., danger of death), all
requests for baptism made by adults or for infants should be
referred to the chaplain of the hospital, who will see that the prescriptions of canon law are observed.

(2)   Even cases of emergency should be referred to the chaplain or to some other priest if one is available. If a priest is not
available, anyone having the use of reason can and should baptize.
(The ordinary method of baptizing is as follows: Water is poured
on the head in such a way that it will flow on the skin, and not
merely on the hair; and while the water is being poured these words
are pronounced: I baptize you in the Name of the Father, and of
the Son, and of the Holy Ghost. The water will more easily flow
on the skin if it is poured on the forehead. The same person who
pours the water should pronounce the words.

(3)   When emergency baptism is conferred, the fact should
be noted on the patient's chart, and the chaplain should be notified
as soon as possible so that he can properly record it.

(4)   It is the mind of the Church that the sick should have the
widest possible liberty to receive the sacraments frequently. The
generous cooperation of the entire hospital staff and personnel is
requested for this purpose.

(5)   While providing the sick abundant opportunity to receive
Holy Communion, there should be no interference with the perfect
freedom of the faithful according to the mind of the Church to
communicate or not to communicate, and moreover there should
be no pressure exerted that might lead to sacrilegious Communions.

---

[1] Barton, R. T.: The Influence of Pregnancy on Otosclerosis. *New England
Journal of Medicine, 233*:433-436 (Oct. 11) 1945.

(6)   Those in danger of death are not obliged to keep the Eucharistic fast. Regarding other privileges available to the sick and hospital personnel, the chaplain or some other priest should be consulted.

(7)   Sufficient privacy should be provided for confession in wards and semi-private rooms, or the patient moved elsewhere for confession, if this is possible.

(8)   When possible, one who is critically ill should receive Holy Viaticum and Extreme Unction while in full possession of his rational faculties. *The chaplain must, therefore, be notified by the physician as soon as an illness is diagnosed as critical.*

(9)   Major parts of the body should be buried in a cemetery when it is reasonably possible to do so. Moreover, the members of Catholicism should, if possible, be buried in blessed ground.

(10)   When burial is not reasonably possible, the burning of such members is permissible.

(11)   When there is a sufficient reason for doing so, a fetus may be retained for laboratory study and observation. It may not, however, be preserved in membranes unless so obviously dead that baptism would be of no avail.

(12)   When sanitation or some similarly serious reason demands it, a fetus may be burned.

(13)   Aside from the cases just indicated, every fetus, regardless of the degree of maturity it has reached, must be suitably buried in a cemetery.

Role of the Physician   The Catholic Church teaches the Catholic physician that his first duty is to acquire a full and competent knowledge of the science and art of medicine and maintain it. Secondly, he must become familiar with the Catholic Medico-Moral Code and follow it. Furthermore, he should give each case the attention due the patient, including the use of consultants when indicated. He is expected to keep all knowledge secret which comes to him in the exercise of his profession, with four special exceptions. These are when it is necessary to disclose the secret in order to avert serious injury to the State, a third party, the person confiding the secret, or the doctor himself. Finally, a Catholic doctor is expected to follow the religious prescriptions at the time of a patient's death, such as calling the priest for the Last Sacrament, etc.

The ecclesiastical canons contain many and various prescriptions concerning lay physicians, which are enumerated by Ferraris (*Bibliotheca Canonica,* Rome: 1889). Thus, physicians are warned that they must endeavor to persuade their patients to make sacramental confession of their sins. St. Pius V decreed that no physician should receive the doctorate unless he took oath not to visit a sick person longer than three days without calling a confessor, unless there was some reasonable excuse. If he violated his oath, he fell under excommunication.

The canons also declare that when a physician is paid by the public community, he is bound to treat ecclesiastics gratis, though the bishop may allow them to make voluntary contributions. Physicians who prescribe remedies involving infractions of the Decalogue, are themselves guilty of grave sin. This is also the case if they experiment on a sick person with unknown medicines, unless all hope has been given up and there is at least a possibility of doing them good. Physicians are to be reminded that they have no dispensing power concerning the fast and abstinence prescribed by the Church. They may, however, give their prudent judgment as to whether a sick person, owing to grave danger or inconvenience to his health, is obliged by the ecclesiastical precept. They are warned that, if they declare unnecessarily that a person, owing to grave danger or inconvenience to health a person is not obliged to fast, they themselves commit grave sin.

They also sin mortally if they attempt, without being forced by necessity, to cure a serious illness, when they are aware that through their own culpable ignorance or inexperience, they may be the cause of grave harm to the patient.

The canons further state, "Physicians who are assigned to the care of convents of nuns should be not less than fifty years of age, and younger practitioners are not to be employed unless those of the prescribed age are not obtainable. When they have the ordinary care of nuns, they are to have general license to enter the cloister, even at night in cases of great urgency. They are not, however, to be alone with the patient."

Father O'Donnell outlines in *Morals in Medicine* the following procedures in cases of known or suspected impotence. The doctor should be aware of these in caring for Catholic patients:

(1) *Before Marriage:* The doctor will sometime see patients who are contemplating marriage and with whom there is some question of impotence. In these instances, the physician should—
a) *If Impotence is certain:* It is the doctor's duty to inform the patient of this and indicate the impossibility of contracting a valid marriage.
b) *If Impotence is doubtful:* If the doctor is not certain that his patient is impotent but has reason to suspect it, he should advise the patient to clear the matter through the ecclesiastical authorities.
c) *If Impotence is temporary:* The doctor may inform the patient of his obligation to correct surgically or by some other legitimate way the impotence before marriage is contemplated.

(2) *After Marriage:* The physician should—
a) *If Impotence is doubtful:* They may attempt marital intercourse until it is certain that it cannot be performed properly.
b) *If Impotence is certain:* The doctor should advise them to consult their parish priest. If the impotence cannot be corrected, and the parties are in good faith and do not know of the impediment, and if separation is morally impossible; or if the priest believes that, if told of the invalidity of their marriage, they will not separate and will thus be knowingly committing fornication, he may leave them in good faith, in some cases.

If the impotence exists in only one party, and they do separate, even though the marriage was invalid, the other party is not free to marry until after an ecclesiastical declaration of nullity.

The non-Catholic physician occasionally finds difficulty in accepting a few of the Church rules. However, if he is privileged to use a Catholic hospital, it seems reasonable that he be expected to conduct himself according to Medico-Moral Code while working in that hospital. It is not reasonable, however, to expect him to follow these precepts in his office or away from the hospital, unless the patient being treated is of the Roman Catholic faith and requests it.[1]

---

[1] Book Reviews: *J.A.M.A., 164*:503 (May 25) 1957.

Mind Cure   Divine healing is still a large part of Catholicism in parts of the world and the use of relics is popular too. Among the most celebrated of relic shrines is that in honor of St. Anne de Beaupre, at Beaupre, Canada. The chapel was founded in 1658. On the very day of dedication the patron saint is said to have shown her favor by healing of rheumatism a man who was in the act of depositing three stones in the foundation of the edifice. From that day to this, a continuous stream of miracles has reportedly manifested the divine favor. It is said that huge pyramids of crutches, walking sticks, bandages and other appliances may be seen on either side of the main entrances, left by those who, having prayed to the saint, have gone away cured.

Since disease is considered a natural cause, Catholics believe that cures may be obtained from God and that special efficacy is attached to their prayers when joined with those of the Blessed Virgin Mary or the Saints. To preclude charges of "mental healing," however, the Church does not accept cures as "official miracles" which involve nervous or hysterical illnesses. It requires for official approval that the cure be irrefutable, i.e., a before and after medical case history, that it be instantaneous or at least obviously faster than nature's usual speed, and/or it involve the restoration of a withered or missing member of the body.

As to psychiatry, the conflict has been given much publicity. The Church took sharp exception to Freud's statement that God was a mere "father-image" invented by man and that religion was a compulsion neurosis.[1] Many theologians felt that his teachings endangered the freedom of the will. However, recently Pope Pius XII publicly approved psychotherapy as one of the weapons of the armory of modern healers, provided "the truths established by reason and by faith and the obligatory precepts of ethics" are observed. Anderson[2] has summarized the Roman Catholic attitude as follows:

"Freudian psychoanalysis has not won the universal support of religious groups because certain Freudian principles threaten tra-

---

[1] Hogan, B. W.: Psychiatry and Religion. *The Linacre Quarterly*, 22:79-85 (Aug.) 1955.

[2] Anderson, G. C.: Conflicts Between Psychiatry and Religion. *J.A.M.A.*, 155: 335-338 (May 22) 1954.

ditional moral and theological concepts. But Freudian psycho-analysis is only one facet of psychiatry. There is a growing appre-ciation within religious circles of the contributions psychiatric research is providing. Theological schools are beginning to intro-duce courses relating these psychiatric insights to religious teach-ings and doctrines. Psychiatry is shedding light on the nature of the unconscious; this fact is important to theologians and students of behavior. A better understanding of the unconscious provides opportunities for the restudy of the theological doctrine of the free-dom of the will. The psychosomatic viewpoint in medicine, enlight-ened by psychiatry, suggests opportunities for religious groups in guiding people toward healthy mental responses, thus aiding a person toward good health physically. Certain psychiatric practices such as lobotomy raise moral questions that need to be examined before religious groups can give complete approval to such prac-tices. The major areas of disagreement between psychiatry and religion concern philosophical attitudes and beliefs. Most of the basic tenets of religion are not invalidated by the contentions of psychiatry; however, there are real differences that need to be resolved. But there is a need for theologians to restudy certain tra-ditional attitudes in the light of psychiatric discoveries. Doctrinal differences also need to be resolved. Psychiatry too must re-examine some of its most cherished concepts before it can expect the total support of all groups working in the field of mental health. Psy-chiatry is not irreligious, for it aims to produce or restore good health. However, certain psychiatric techniques may conflict with traditional religious beliefs. Religion and psychiatry, working together, have much to contribute in the search for health."

Supplementary Reading

Bonnar, A.: *The Catholic Doctor.* London, Burns, Oates and Wash-bourne, 1948.

Catholic Encyclopedia: New York, Encyclopedia Press, 1913.

Dawson, G. G.: *Healing: Pagan and Christian.* New York, Macmillan, 1935.

Gemelli, Agostino: *Psychoanalysis Today.* New York, Kennedy, 1955.

Good, F. L., and Kelly, O. F.: *Marriage, Morals, and Medical Ethics.* New York, Kennedy, 1951.

Hastings, J., Ed.: *Encyclopaedia of Religion and Ethics.* New York, Scribner, 1910.

Hayes, E. J., Hayer, P. J., and Kelly, D. E.: *Moral Handbook of Nursing.* New York, Macmillan, 1956.

Liotta, M. A.: *Connection Between Religion and Medicine.* New York, J. J. Little and Ives Co., 1935.

Messenger, E. C.: *Two In One Flesh.* Westminister, Newman Press, 1948.

Misiak, H.: Psychosomatic Medicine and Religion. *Catholic World,* February, 1953, pp. 342-345.

Odenwald, R. P., and Vander Veldt, J. H.: *Psychiatry and Catholicism.* New York, McGraw-Hill, 1952.

Sheen, F. J.: *Three To Get Married.* New York, Appleton-Century-Crofts, 1951.

Smith, G. D.: *The Teaching of the Catholic Church.* London, Burns, Oates and Washbourne, 1948.

Walsh, J. J.: *Religion and Health.* Boston, Little, Brown & Co., 1920.

PROTESTANTISM

History   The leader of the Reformation and founder of the Reformed Church was an Augustinian monk, Martin Luther, who in 1517 set off a reaction which again split Christianity. His main objection at the outset was to the sale of "indulgences," and he at first demanded reform with no intention of leaving the Western Church. However, by 1529 the break was beyond repair and the term "protestant" had been applied as a generic name to the Reformed and Evangelical Churches.

The fire of the Reformation broke out in many countries with different leaders and a variety of beliefs. One of these, Huldreich Zwingli, was a Catholic priest in Switzerland who led the Reform in that country and who was killed in a religious civil war between the Evangelical Swiss and the five Romanist Cantons. Another, John Calvin, was a scholar born and educated in France, but who moved to Geneva and there became an influential reformer. His theology is the basis for such denominations as the Presbyterian Church, founded by Calvin's disciple, John Knox. Still another contemporary of these men was Menno Simons, a Catholic priest whose reformed teachings led to the founding of the Swiss Brethren, the Mennonite Brethren in Christ, and other Mennonite denominations.

The origins of other Protestant denominations are more complex. The anabaptists, for example, were groups formed during the Reformation in Germany largely, and were the ecclesiastical ancestors of the Baptists of today. The latter denomination was founded in 1611 in England and was introduced into America by Roger Williams. The Brethren bodies in America usually represent vestiges of the German Baptist movement.

The Church of England is another Christian church which claims apostolic succession. It is said to be both Catholic (universal) and Protestant (reformed). The split with Rome was aggravated by Henry VIII, who desired a divorce. However, the actual cause of the separation from Rome in 1534 A.D. was of long-standing and largely similar to that of the Eastern Church. It came as a protest to the Bishop of Rome's authority, inasmuch as it claimed to have always been more British than Roman. The Anglican Communion in America is the Protestant Episcopal Church. The Congregational Church is the outgrowth of a splinter group of the Church of England which migrated to America and later separated from the Anglican Communion. Similarly the Methodist Church was founded in 1738 by an Anglican priest, John Wesley, whose intention was not to leave the Church of England but to form societies within it. The Bishop of London refused to ordain Wesley's ministers, and as a result the Methodist Episcopal Church was organized separately in America in 1784.

Quakerism sprang up in England in the Seventeenth century, founded by George Fox. The Religious Society of Friends, as it is formally known, is basically a Protestant denomination, although they consider themselves a "third way" of Christianity.

Also, not strictly "Christian" in the sense that they do not worship Jesus Christ as "Lord and God," the Unitarian Church may be placed in the Protestant category because of its origin and general beliefs. The Unitarian movement was founded by Francis David, Faustus Socinus and Michael Servetus in the sixteenth century as a protest against the dogma of the trinity and the development of "Christology." Branches of this church were among the first churches in America. It is significant of the temper of the time of the Reformation to point out that Servetus was ordered burned to death by John Calvin over a theological quibble. Servetus, of course, was the great anatomist who nearly anticipated Harvey's discovery of the circulation of the blood. He was, too, an intense and independent biblicist and thereby drew the wrath of the zealous Calvin.

The Hutterites are a small Protestant sect found in the Dakotas and Montana of the United States and Alberta and Manitoba Provinces in Canada. They originated in Europe in 1762, suffering through the years from much persecution, and fleeing from Europe to Russia to the United States and finally Canada. Today, this group is prosperous and productive, living together in a communal type of organization. They are of interest primarily from the standpoint of human biology, because no economic pressure exists among them for pregnancy limitation. The colony provides equally for all families, regardless of size or industry of the main provider. The birth of another child in no way penalizes the standard of living; the communal carpenter simply saws another bed. The family may be given an apartment with an extra room and if the mother needs additional household help, a relative or neighbor comes in to share the work. The colony pays the medical bills. As a consequence, they have represented an ideal opportunity to study human fecundity.[1]

Nature of Disease   Belief in the "original sin" as a cause of man's suffering and illness is held by only a few Protestant denominations. Others, such as the Unitarians and the Disciples of Christ, reject it outright. However, most of the churches hold that God may intercede and restore health through "divine healing," in conjunction with medical science or sometimes apart from medical supervision. Disease is generally not considered a punishment nor is it considered unreal,[2] although there are some exceptions to this amongst the Calvinist-inclined.

Luther taught that many physical ills have their origin in spiritual anxiety; sorrow, temptation, guilt and fear were regarded as spiritual states that needed the cure of prayer and spiritual consultation with a pastor. Occasionally, the Calvinistic doctrine of

---

[1] Eaton, J. W. and Mayer, A. J.: The Social Biology of Very High Fertility Among the Hutterites: The Demography of a Unique Population. *Human Biol., 25*:206, 1953.

[2] Hiltner, S.: Religion and Health. *American Scholar*, July, 1946, p. 327.

predestination is still reflected in some patients thinking that their condition is ordained by God and that they should resign themselves to His will. However, as Dr. Goodspeed has pointed out, generally these Christians believe in the love and care of God and in His interest in the well-being of the individual.[1]

Diet The Protestant groups born during the Reformation abandoned all of the Jewish and Roman Catholic dietary rules. Many of them subsequently became strongly opposed to alcoholic beverages and tobacco smoking. There is in this latter regard some diversity of opinion, however.

Throughout Protestantism one finds only a few dietary ideas that are generally unorthodox and they do not represent an official belief. Some still partially accept the Biblical stigma of pork, for example. Another interesting concept is proposed by the Rev. Charlie Shedd[2] for the management of obesity through prayer. He states, "The spiritual approach to reducing is a sure road to healing your obesity, permanently."

Therapy Many of these denominations have pioneered in bringing the church and medical science together. As Henry J. Cadbury[3] has pointed out, for example, the Quakers led in the improved treatment of the insane when they founded the Retreat at York, England, in 1779. Protestant hospitals are prominent all over the world today.

It is difficult to give a single Protestant position on most points of morality because of the diverse opinions within Christian Protestantism. Generally, though, contemporary belief is that the sex motives of procreation and love or pleasure are of equal importance. Virginity and celibacy are rejected as false goals arising from the corruption of Christianity by Hellenistic dualism.[4] Most of the Protestant bodies take liberal and cooperative attitudes toward medicine. Birth control is not thought of as a sin. They take the position that it should not be abused and is especially worthwhile

---

[1] Goodspeed, E. J.: *A Modern Apocrypha.* Boston, Beacon, 1957.

[2] Shedd, C.: *Pray Your Weight Away.* New York, Lippincott, 1957.

[3] Cadbury, Henry J.: *George Fox's Book of Miracles.* Cambridge, Cambridge University Press, 1947.

[4] Cole, W. G.: *Sex in Christianity and Psychoanalysis.* New York, Oxford University Press, 1955.

for certain health reasons. The Hutterites, however, consider contraception as an act of murder. Probably, the recent statement of the Methodist General Conference best summarizes the general Protestant belief. It states, "We believe that planned parenthood, practiced in Christian conscience, may fulfill rather than violate the will of God."

It is primarily in the areas of sex that Protestant belief differs from Roman Catholic. Most Protestant hospitals follow the same general code as that listed for the Catholic Hospital Association, with certain exceptions such as the baptism and Extreme Unction rules and the regulations concerning therapeutic abortion (Catholic priests say there is no such thing), artificial insemination, contraception, etc.

Very little has been written on the ethics of medical practice by Protestant leaders, but one of the most recent books covering a limited number of ethical problems is that of the Rev. Joseph Fletcher.[1] This discussion is based on a personalist philosophy which is not necessarily representative of all Protestant groups. Similarly, his conclusions probably do not represent the thinking of the majority of Protestant theologians. He argues for "our human rights (certain conditions being satisfied) to use contraceptives, to seek insemination anonymously from a donor, to be sterilized, and to receive a merciful death from a medically competent euthanasiast." His argument for semiadoption[2] is effective, but the discussion of "mercy killing" largely fails to appreciate the various medical aspects of the problem.[3] Finally, Rev. Fletcher contends that it is the patient's right to know the truth regarding his health.

All of the Protestant groups reject the belief in the efficacy of relics and emphasize the therapeutic value of the Christian virtues, such as faith, love and forgiveness. They do not unanimously con-

---

[1] Fletcher, Jos.: *Morals and Medicine.* Princeton, Princeton University Press, 1954.

[2] A preferred term for artificial insemination, proposed by Kleegman and Cary, demonstrating that one partner of the marriage is definitely the parent, and the second partner has "adopted the child" produced by this treatment. See Simmons, F. A.: Human Fertility. *New England J. Med., 255:*1189 (Dec. 20) 1956.

[3] Smith, C. A.: The Doomed Infant and Child. *Rhode Island Med. J.* (Sept.) 1956.

demn suicide, although they teach that the body is "God's temple" and should be properly cared for.

Role of the Physician   The American Protestant Hospital Association is an organization somewhat analogous to the American Catholic Hospital Association, except that it is basically a church liaison organization providing a trained chaplaincy and in no way dictates rules and regulations for medical conduct.[1] For this reason, the physician seldom has differences with the Protestant chaplaincy so long as he practices according to the standard of the community.

Most Protestant groups believe that God works through the physician in response to prayer. They recognize that the Apostle Luke was a physician and that God therefore holds a place for the doctor in caring for the sick.

Incidentally, the Emmanuel Movement was a group of historical importance in that it attempted to effectively bring together religion and medicine. It was inaugurated by the Rev. Elwood Worcester and was popular for some time in Boston among medical and religious leaders. The approach to healing was both scientific and religious with both pastor and physician ministering to the patient. The system never became popular, because generally the patient had faith in one or the other (either religion or medicine) and usually did not want both.

Mind Cure   The early Protestant Church had many faith healers, such as the Lutheran pastor, John Blumhardt, who practiced the "laying on of the hands." He later established an institution for religious healing not unlike the shrine of Lourdes. Many of the early American sects emphasized healing too, especially the Shaker leader, "Mother Ann." Today, the beliefs in divine healing vary greatly from the restrained attitude of the orthodox Protestant, such as the Anglican priest Rev. John Maillard, to the "Healing Waters" of Oral Roberts, who employs "anointed handkerchiefs," etc.

Protestantism has never been as critical of psychiatry as the Roman Catholic Church.[2] In fact, many of their clergymen have

---

1 Scherzer, Carl J.: *The Church and Healing.* Philadelphia, The Westminister Press, 1950.

2 Bier, W. C.: Sigmund Freud and The Faith. *America,* p. 196 (Nov. 17) 1956.

taken up a certain amount of the terminology.[1] They believe that prayer may have a therapeutic effect, if only because it enables people to verbalize their reflections and wishes. The same is considered true of hymns, as recognized by Luther. Finally, they believe the psychological value of religion is that of providing an individual's life with unity and meaning.

One of the most outstanding Protestant clergymen as far as the study of religion and psychology is concerned is Dr. Leslie D. Weatherhead of London. He states, "At our present state of development any attitude of mind which regards as unnecessary the doctor, surgeon, dentist, nurse, masseur or other qualified worker on the physical level stands self-condemned." "No amount of love, or positive-thinking, or denial of the existence of evil will take a spinter out of an eye."[2]

At the same time, Weatherhead points out, man is not mere body. The influence of the mind has been emphasized again and again. His opinion is that Freudian psychoanalysis is too time-consuming, too expensive for all but the very few. The use of drugs often helps, but it is of questionable lasting value. "In my opinion, all methods used so far will seem to be, judged by future standards, a blundering and groping tinkering with the mind, as clumsy and intolerably tedious as the early surgical operations appear now in the eyes of the efficient modern surgeon," he says.

Religion on the other hand, Weatherhead writes, has lost a supernatural gift of healing which it claimed in the first century and he calls for the churches and their members to recover "the lost art of healing through the direct activity of God." "Let the Church have its psychological clinics. I strongly recommend this. But Christ did not send out His Apostles to be psychologists and doctors, but to be the spearheads of fellowships made one through a discipline to prayer and corporate worship. Let the Church support all that is being done to heal men through every known scientific means, but let it not be bluffed into supposing that that is the healing work it is called to do," concludes Weatherhead.

---

[1] Weatherhead, L. D.: Christian Faith and Psychotherapy. *Religion in Life*, No. 4, 1952, p. 483.

[2] Weatherhead, L. D.: *Psychology, Religion and Healing.* New York, Abingdon Press, 1955.

Two interesting points are made by this church leader regarding this use of religion for healing. He contends that this is legiti mate only up to a point. "It breaks down if the patient only regards religion as he regards other means of getting better." Furthermore, he states, "I do not mean that Christian fellowship is able to cure anything. In my view, there are situations where God has decreed that the relevant way of cooperating with Him is that of medicine, surgery, psychology, or other scientific technique."

Supplementary Reading

Are you looking for God? Clinic where Doctors and Clergymen join hands. *American Magazine,* October, 1947, p. 21.

Braden, C. S.: Health, Wealth and Faith. *Christian Century,* January 19, 1944, p. 78.

Conditions of Medical Responsibility. *Review of Religion,* March, 1949, p. 241.

Dicks, R. L.: *God and Health.* New York, 1947.

Ferm, U.: *Pictorial History of Protestantism.* New York, Philosophical Library, 1957.

Goldstein, K.: Idea of Disease and Therapy. *Review of Religion,* March, 1949, p. 229.

Heim, K.: *Christian Faith and Natural Science.* New York, Torchbooks, 1957.

Julian, F. B.: Influence of religion on the progress of medicine. *Hibbert Journal,* April, 1953, p. 254.

Kemp, P.: *Healing Ritual.* London, Faber and Faber, 1935.

Liotta, M. A.: *The Connection Between Religion and Medicine.* New York, J. J. Little and Ives Co., 1935.

Niebuhr, R.: Sex Standards in America. *Christianity and Crisis,* May, 1948.

Physical Methods in Psychiatry and Spiritual Healing. *Spectator,* May 21, 1954, p. 610.

Psychiatry for Pastors. *Time,* October 26, 1953, p. 69.

Tilich, P.: Psychotherapy and a Christian interpretation of human nature. *Review of Religion,* March, 1949, p. 264.

Vanderweldt, J.: Religion and Mental Health. *Mental Hygiene,* April, 1951, p. 177.

V

RELIGIONS OF AMERICAN ORIGIN

Most of the religious bodies included in this group are of the Christian Protestant tradition, although not connected with the Reformation directly. Some of the churches, however, resulted from a "protestant" movement against the Protestant beliefs, such as the Churches of Christ ("Christians") and the Disciples of Christ ("Disciples"), which are schisms of the Presbyterian and Baptist Churches.

The Christians led by Barton W. Stone and the Disciples ("Campbellites") founded by Thomas Campbell and his son, Alexander, joined forces in 1832 and remained together for about sixty years, but today they are divided again. They are the largest indigenous American religious groups, and their doctrines are similar to those described in the Christian Protestant section, insofar as medical practice is concerned.

Other American churches are simply Negro branches of various denominations, such as African Orthodox (Episcopalian), National Baptist Convention, African Methodist Episcopal, etc. Their beliefs and doctrines are similar to the parent group. Churches such as the various Evangelistic Associations, Foursquare Gospel, etc., are of the general Protestant belief. Another group of American religions has been set aside in a separate category, not because of their size or origin but because they represent a pragmatic thought, which departs from most Christian doctrine of the past. William James has named them the "Religions of Healthy-Mindedness."

LATTER-DAY-SAINTS

History   The Church of Jesus Christ of Latter-Day-Saints became a legal entity in 1830 at Fayette, Seneca County, New York. Ten years prior to that time Joseph Smith, the founder, experienced his divine revelation near Palmyra, New York. This led to his receipt of the gold engraved record plates prepared by Mormon comprising a condensation of: The plates of Nephi, Ether, the brass plates of Laban, and the records of other ancient American historians. The message on these was recorded and published by Smith in 1830.[1]

Membership quickly increased and so did opposition. The main body first moved to Ohio, then to Missouri, then to Illinois. In each location they were persecuted, and in Carthage, Illinois, in 1844 Joseph Smith was killed by an armed mob. In 1847 his successor, Brigham Young, led the members into the valley of the Great Salt Lake where the headquarters of the church was established. Today there are over 1,300,000 "Mormons" as they have been nicknamed throughout the world.

The "Mormon" church is Christian but not Protestant in that it does not protest against any church, and it honors Joseph Smith, Brigham Young and all the succeeding presidents of the church including the present one, in a similar manner as it honors the prophets of the Old and New Testaments.[2] The practice of polygamy is now prohibited with the penalty of excommunication.

Nature of Disease   Although Brigham Young taught that sickness and disease appeared "if we defile ourselves," this concept is no longer used to explain all of one's maladies. Young[3] emphasized the importance of proper eating, out-of-door living and exercise to maintain health.

Today the church's attitude is that sickness is real, sometimes inevitable or unavoidable, but to be cured or endured according to God's will.

Diet   The code of health and conduct given in 1833 was known as the "Word of Wisdom." It disapproves of the use of tobacco, alcoholic beverages, and "hot drinks" (meaning tea and coffee). Brigham Young, in talking on "Eating for Health," advised

---

[1] Smith, Joseph: *The Book of Mormon.* Salt Lake City, The Church of Latter-Day Saints, 1920.

[2] Smith, Joseph: *Teachings of the Prophet Joseph Smith.* Salt Lake City, Deseret News Press, 1938.

[3] Widtsoe, John A., ed: *Discourses of Brigham Young.* Salt Lake City, Deseret Book Company, 1925.

drinking "good, clear mountain water," eating fruits and vegetables, avoiding pork and eating moderately of simple food. (There is no prohibition against pork if it is properly cooked.)

Furthermore, he advised that children be given a limited amount of meat, especially fat meat, but that they should have "milk, bread, water and potatoes and other vegetables."

Role of the Physician   Young once said, "Instead of calling for the doctor you should administer to them (the sick) by the laying on of hands and anointing with oil, and give them mild food and herbs and medicines that you understand." He believed that God would direct the management of the sick if called upon.

Today "Mormons" call upon the physician freely and pray that the Lord will bless the sick through him. It is, however, the practice of the Latter-Day Saints to call upon the elders to lay their hands upon the head of the patient and give him a blessing before he goes into surgery, requesting that the Lord's healing influence might attend him and guide and direct the surgeons and others assisting in the operation.

Therapy   Among "Mormons" there is prohibition against the use of stimulants such as benzedrine, and against the use of narcotics, except when prescribed by a duly licensed physician. Great importance is attached to living "out of doors" and vigorous exercise. There is no prejudice against modern surgery, antibiotics, etc. They have always advocated the rearing of large families, and birth control is contrary to their teachings except when the attending physician feels that the health of the mother would be impaired by continuous child bearing. In the case of childbirth, if a choice definitely must be made between the life of the mother and the life of the child, the mother should be given first consideration.

Mind Cure   The "Mormon" church has no open differences with psychiatry, psychoanalysis and psychosurgery when practiced by competent physicians. Brigham Young did emphasize the relationship between exercise and mental vigor stating, "My mind becomes tired, and perhaps some of yours do. If so, go and exercise your bodies." "Many persons are so constituted, that if you put them in a parlor, keep a good fire for them, furnish them tea, cake, sweet meats, etc., and nurse them tenderly, soaking their feet, and putting them to bed, they will die in a short time; but throw them into snow banks, and they will live a great many years."

Supplementary Reading

Bennion, Lowell L.: *The Religion of the Latter-Day Saints.* Salt Lake City, Latter-Day Saints Department of Education, 1940.

Durham, G. Homer: *Joseph Smith, Prophet-Statesman.* New York, Bookcraft Company, 1944.

Evans, John: *Leadership of Joseph Smith.* M.I.A. Manual, 1934-1935.

Houf, Horace T.: *What Religion Is and Does.* New York, Harper, 1935.

Kinney, Bruce: *Mormonism.* New York, Fleming H. Revell Company, 1912.

Widtsoe, John A.: *The Program of the Church.* Salt Lake City, Latter-Day Saints Department of Education, 1936.

——————: *A Rational Theology.* Salt Lake City, Deseret Book Company, 1937.

——————: *An Understandable Religion.* Salt Lake City, Zion's Printing Company, 1944.

——————, and Leah D.: *The Word of Wisdom.* Salt Lake City, Zion's Printing Company, 1948.

JEHOVAH'S WITNESSES

History   In 1870, Charles Taze Russell organized a group for the systematic study of the Bible. He was later chosen by the members to be editor of a monthly magazine called *Zion's Watch Tower and Herald of Christ's Presence.* In 1881, Zion's Watch Tower Tract Society was established as an administrative agency, and was incorporated on December 13, 1884, in Allegheny County, Pennsylvania, thus giving the Society legal life. Its original corporate name, Zion's Watch Tower Tract Society, was changed in 1896, by court-sanctioned amendment, to its present name, "Watch Tower Bible and Tract Society," but the name, Jehovah's Witnesses, was not used until 1931.

"Judge" Rutherford, Russell's successor, was a Missouri lawyer who had occasionally sat as a circuit court judge.[1] He wrote tirelessly and popularized the denominational beliefs. One of these precepts was to "not advise on health matters except as they may involve Scriptural issues. Fanaticism in health matters is unwise, and absorption in health fads is a form of introversion that keeps the mind on oneself, which is conducive to neither physical nor spiritual health. Sweeping claims for cures by this or that system are always suspect. Each individual differs. Moderation is usually beneficial."

Witnesses believe there is only the "one faith" as expressed by Paul and that one is as practical for our day as it was for the Hebrews and Greeks of the Bible.[2]

Nature of Disease   Jehovah's Witnesses believe that all the sickness that has entered the earth resulted from the original violation of God's law. Likewise today, "sickness and disease are due to some violation of God's law concerning physical well-being. They are not due to the direct touch of Satan. Various ones of us may inherit tendencies to certain bodily ailments, and these may appear after certain causes lead them to develop and break out. Say a plague is sweeping the land. A worldling with a healthy constitution may go through it unaffected, whereas a faithful Christian may be laid low with it and die or have a hard time recovering. The reason for this may lie entirely in the weaker physical frame and in not knowing what precautions to take against becoming infected. So these are natural, physical processes which operate in any and all persons regardless of one's faith. It would be unreasonable to blame the Devil directly. Sickness, diseases and accidents have their normal causes. These causes produce the same results in the lives of unconsecrated worldlings. So sickness, malignant maladies, accidents, and old age may be expected to take their usual course among devoted Christians the same as among the rest of mankind." So states the *Watchtower*, May 15, 1951, pages 297 to 299.

---

[1] Mead, F. S.: *Handbook of Denominations.* New York, Abingdon Press, 1956.

[2] Henschel, M. G.: Who Are Jehovah's Witnesses? Pp. 58-64 of *A Guide to the Religions of America.* Edited by Leo Rosten. New York, Simon and Schuster, 1955.

Diet   There are no rules as to special food habits; in fact, Mr. Russell originally stated that the group was not concerned with diet and that members were entitled to eat what they chose.[1] Judge Rutherford has added that all food is "religiously clean," yet some Jewish Witnesses of orthodox background still follow the traditional dietary laws.

Therapy   No prohibition is made of the use of drugs, although again there is the idea that "drugging" can be overdone and that moderation and common sense should be the rule. As stated in the *Watchtower*, "We leave it up to each individual to choose his own type of treatment. Some may favor surgery, some medicines, some diet, and some may prefer other forms of treatment. One illness may require surgery, another may call for dieting. Also, the treatment that helps one may be of no aid or even be detrimental to another. So let each one go to those who are trained in the treatment of his choice."

Jehovah's Witnesses, as a group, do not believe in blood transfusions,[2] but allow each member the right to decide for himself what he can conscientiously do. This concept is based on the idea that blood is sacred and that the Biblical injunction of not eating blood means that transfusions are forbidden. Beside the theological objections, they point out that blood transfusions can be dangerous, and actually injurious. Therefore, they have recently championed the use of blood substitutes. However, this belief against transfusions has been subjected to a legal test in the famous Labrenz case in Chicago. It was ruled in that instance that the parents of the child were "technically negligent" in forbidding a transfusion for the daughter and ordered that she be put in court custody and transfused.

The attitude toward birth control is that the purpose of marriage is the rearing of children, but they regard birth control as an entirely personal matter.

---

[1] Stroup, H. H.: *The Jehovah's Witnesses*. New York, Columbia University Press, 1945.

[2] Blood Transfusions—Jehovah's Witnesses. *J.A.M.A., 163*:660-661 (Feb. 23) 1957.

Role of the Physician   In this regard, the *Watchtower* comments, "When we fall sick or certain ailments come on us with old age, we may turn to natural methods of cure or medical remedies. We may resort to doctors or whatever school seems to us to be the best. We may go to sanatoria or to hospitals or have a surgical operation. Such curative methods are not barred to a Christian of faith. We need not delay the proper treatment or care of ourselves by praying and waiting upon miraculous divine healing." In the treatment of a Witness, therefore, the physician need only to settle the issue of blood transfusions when indicated and he will generally find the patient otherwise cooperative.

Mind Cure   The belief in modern-day miracle healing is rejected and is considered to have ceased at the time of the twelve apostles' death. Jehovah's Witnesses believe that the gift of miracle-healing was made by Jesus Christ to His disciples and was never passed on to others.

They advise against "having anything to do with hypnosis or hypnotic therapy," as it requires the patient to "surrender his will to another." This is considered immoral, "even when surrendered temporarily," because "the Christian has agreed to do only Jehovah's will."

A somewhat similar attitude is held toward psychiatry and psychotherapy. The magazine, *Awake,* states, "The record of Christians for the past nineteen centuries proves that men have been able to make their minds over, let go of their former vices, and 'put on the new personality' which was created according to God's will in true righteousness and loving kindness without resorting to psychiatry."

Supplementary Reading

Blood for a Baby. *Newsweek,* April 30, 1951, p. 25.
Fardon, A. H., and McFarland, H. J.: *Jehovah's Witnesses: Who are They; What do they Teach?* Chicago, Open Court, 1941.
High, S.: Armageddon, Inc. *Saturday Evening Post,* September 14, 1940.
Law and the Life. *Time,* April 30, 1951, pp. 84-85.
Peddlers of Paradise. *American Magazine,* November, 1940.

Putman, C. E.: *Jehovah's Witnesses.* Randleman, North Carolina, The Author, n.d.

Russell, C. T.: *Studies in the Scriptures,* Series I. Brooklyn, International Bible Students Association, Watch Tower Bible and Tract Society, 1925.

Shields, T. T.: *Russellism, Rutherfordism; The Teachings of the International Bible Students Alias Jehovah's Witnesses in the Light of the Holy Scriptures.* Grand Rapids, n.p., 1934.

Transfusion Case to be Fought by Witnesses. *Christian Century,* June 13, 1951, p. 701.

ADVENTIST

History   This ultra-conservative branch of the Protestant body was not formally organized until 1863; yet because of its own medical schools and hospitals, it has contributed greatly to medical practice and thought in various parts of America. Their basic hygienic tenet is that the body is the "temple of the Holy Ghost" and should, therefore, be given the proper care. The dead, according to this doctrine, are awaiting the resurrection in an unconscious state, and will be bodily resurrected on the last day with immortality for the righteous and extinction by fire for the wicked.[1]

The Seventh-Day Adventist sanitariums were conceived as more than mere hospitals, but as educational institutions where the patients would be taught their principles of hygiene. Their medical mission and program has contributed to the improvement of the health of backward peoples.

Nature of Disease   "Pain, sickness, and death are the penalties of transgression" of our first parents (The Original Sin). Often punishment comes to the sinner because of his own sin, however Seventh-Day Adventists believe that not all sickness comes from sins committed. Jesus refers to this in the case of the congenital blind (John 9:1-3) and in the case of Job, God severely reprimanded those who suggested that Job's ailments were the result of some hidden sin or transgression. Adventists hold, therefore, that faith and trust in God are mighty aids in the recovery

---

[1] White, E. G.: *The Great Controversy.* Mountain View, Pacific Press Publishing Association, 1939.

of health, and, when combined with the scientific treatment of disease, they actually bring renewed life to the body as well as the soul.

Diet   Seventh-Day Adventists have ever been of the decided opinion that diet is the key to health and determines largely whether the individual shall be sick or well.

The emphasis in their teaching[1] has been on the eating of fruits, grains, nuts, and vegetables, and the strict avoidance of "flesh foods," meaning meat. Their authorities point out the unfavorable effect of a high protein diet on chronic glomerulo-nephritis, the role of a high cholesterol diet in arteriosclerosis, etc., as being evidence that the eating of meat plays an etiological role in cancer. They, therefore, condemn meat, fish, or shell-fish; but they do eat animal products such as eggs, butter, milk, etc. Cheese, however, is not recommended, but cottage cheese is acceptable. It should be emphasized that while these foods are not recommended, it is not made a "test of fellowship" nor does the use of "flesh foods" bar one from membership in the Seventh-Day Adventist Church.

Therapy   The Seventh-Day Adventist sanitariums were among the first to employ hydrotherapy and electrotherapy. At the same time, the earlier stand was firmly against drugs and medication, but today their physicians use insulin, quinine, antibiotics, etc. Nevertheless, they still hold that the medical profession as a whole is sometimes tempted to depend too much on drugs rather than upon "faith in God and such natural remedies as water, food, sunlight, rest, exercise, and recreation."

The church doctrine discourages the use of tea, coffee, pepper, mustard, hot sauces, tobacco, narcotics, alcohol, and anything else "that injures the body."[2] Fasting is occasionally recommended, although there are no actual fast days in the church.

---

1 Baker, A. L.: *Belief and Work of the Seventh-Day Adventists.* Mountain View, Pacific Press Publishing Association, 1930.

2 Kress, Daniel H.: *The Cigarette As A Physician Sees It.* Mountain View, Pacific Press Publishing Assn., 1942. Thomason, G.: *Science Speaks.* Mountain View, Pacific Press Publishing Assn., 1938. Parrett, O. S.: *Diseases of Food Animals.* Nashville, Southern Publishing Assn., 1951.

Role of the Physician   T. R. Flaiz, M. D., Secretary of the Medical Department of the General Conference of Seventh-Day Adventists, has emphasized their belief that Christ is the "Great Physician," and that He is the true head of the medical profession. The physician is a co-worker with Christ, and should gain His strength and wisdom through prayer. The doctor's personal life and professional life should be exemplary.

In dealing with an Adventist patient, the physician should be aware of their dietary rules and their disapproval of tobacco and alcohol. The doctor is very likely to offend by smoking in the patient's presence.

Mind Cure   The attitude toward psychiatry is one of disapproval only when the patient depends upon the guidance of the psychiatrist rather than God. The concepts of mental health include cultivating a happy, optimistic point of view, avoiding egocentricity, doing good deeds, and prayer. They advance a three-fold approach to psychosomatic problems: "body, mind, and soul," i.e. ministering to the body, using psychotherapy liberally, and not overlooking the spiritual side of man's nature.

Supplementary Reading

Branson, W. H.: Reply to Canright, *The Truth About The Seventh-Day Adventists.* Washington, D. C., Review and Herald Publishing Co., 1933.

Bunch, T. G.: *The Everlasting Gospel.* Loma Linda, California, n.p., 1934.

McCumber, H. O.: *Beginnings of the Seventh-Day Adventist Church in California.* Berkeley, Unpublished Ph.D. Thesis, University of California, 1934.

Nichol, F. D.: *The Midnight Cry.* Washington, Review and Herald Publishing Co., 1935.

Richards, H. M. S.: *New Radio Lectures.* Glendale Academy Press, 1935.

Wearner, A. J.: *Fundamentals of Bible Doctrine.* Angwin, Pacific Union College Press, n.d.

Weber, J. A., Comp.: *Religions and Philosophies in the United States of America.* Los Angeles, Wetzel Publishing Co., 1931.

White, E. G.: *The Story of Patriarchs and Prophets.* Mountain View, Pacific Press Publishing Association, 1947.
——————: *The Ministry of Healing.* Mountain View, Pacific Press Publishing Association, 1942.

VI

RELIGIONS OF HEALTHY-MINDEDNESS

This group of teachings had its origins, as pointed out by William James,[1] in the happiness which a religious belief affords. However, in the past century, the deliberate refusal to think ill of life has been idealized into a systematic cultivation of healthy-mindedness in contrast to the hell-fire theology. The main attack is on "fear" and the "misery-habit" with an emphasis on optimism and the use of the subconscious affirmatively. The facts are that they have stood the pragmatic test on enough occasions that they are a growing and prospering group.[2] Certainly the minimizing of anxieties from fear, remorse, etc. is a favorable device physiologically.

The origin of these "New Thought" groups can be traced back to Phineas Quimby, a clockmaker of Portland, Maine, who studied hypnotism and psychology and decided that a man can change his physical situation by proper thinking. From his impetus in the 1860's, a great variety of sects grew in the United States, England and Canada. Later, various compromises had to be made with medical science. Some, as you shall see in the Christian Science section, have made a minimum of exceptions to the use of divine healing alone, whereas others have come around to the position of working with the physician. The latter is the case with Unity and its related groups.

The truth, of course, is that many members of the Christian Science Church seek medical aid at various times when their "faith is not strong enough alone," or when their religion permits it. Generally too, they make oddly pleasant patients due to their disciplined thinking.

---

[1] James, William: *The Varieties of Religious Experiences: A Study in Human Nature.* New York, Longmans, Green and Co., 1902.

[2] Reed, L. S.: *The Healing Cults.* Chicago, University of Chicago Press, 1946.

Finally, these religions of healthy-mindedness are usually accepted in those countries which have a high standard of public health and thus allow a certain disregard by the individual of contagion prophylaxis. Mrs. Eddy, for example, taught that cows and horses would not become ill unless their human masters injected the animals with belief in disease. On the other hand, Unity does not accept the Mary Baker Eddy concept that disease may be projected into the individual by the improper thinking of someone else. This, Mrs. Eddy called "Malicious Animal Magnetism." When Mr. Eddy died, it was announced that he had died of arsenical poisoning "mentally administered." His wife alleged that the arsenic had been *thought* into him by his enemies. (An autopsy demonstrated that the cause of death was heart disease.) It is the Unity viewpoint that no one else can inject negative ideas into you, that these are your personal creation, if present.

There is a new trend among the Christian Protestant churches to bring some of this teaching into their groups, and such leaders as Dr. Norman Vincent Peale[1] have popularized "positive thinking," stating that "God heals in two ways: through His servants, the practitioners of scientific medicine, and through His servants, the practitioners of sound faith." His ideas that a mass of unhappy thought can produce physical symptoms of disease and that right thinking and living can lead to well-being are not unlike those of the other religions of healthy-mindedness. He and his collaborator, psychiatrist Smiley Blanton,[2] have set up church-sponsored clinics for this religious approach to healing.

The Jewish Science Movement has been mentioned in the section on Judaism. It represents a similar positive-thinking system of spiritual healing, teaching "how to heal oneself and others" and to apply "the principles to overcome worry, conquer fear, subdue anger, and live a joyful, optimistic and serene life." Rabbi Liebman's "Peace of Mind"[3] is not greatly different in aim to this Jewish Science concept.

---

[1] Peale, N. V.: Address at the Inaugural Ceremonies. *J.A.M.A., 158*:1553-1554 (Aug. 27) 1955.

[2] Author of *Love or Perish*. New York, Simon and Schuster, 1956.

[3] Published by Simon and Schuster, 1946.

CHRISTIAN SCIENCE

History   The concepts of this religious group were discovered by Mary Baker Eddy in 1866 and eleven years later her church was formally organized. As applied to health, the principal feature is "the scientific system of divine healing." However, Christian Scientists do not limit their practice to the healing of the sick, but apply their mental and spiritual methods to practically every human need.

Certain terms are important in the exposition of Christian Science. Animal magnetism is the mesmeric action of erroneous belief; Christian Science is its antithesis. Healing is not miraculous but divinely natural; disease is a mental concept dispelled by the introduction of spiritual truth. Heaven is not a locality but "harmony." Hell is "mortal belief, error, lust, remorse, hatred, revenge, sin, sickness, death, suffering, etc.

Nature of Disease   Christian Science draws an absolute distinction between what is real and what is apparent or seeming but unreal. This is extended to the point that disease and death are considered to be unreal and non-existent.[1]

Healing   When ill, the "Scientist" treats himself by dwelling upon the thought that illness has no divine source or origin, that God does not create nor include it, and that "it is therefore spiritually powerless and factually unreal." He affirms the "omnipresence of good, Mind, and denies the power of evil to seize or control his thinking or his body." He dwells upon "pertinent passages which may come to him or which he may seek out by way of concordances from the Holy Bible and Mrs. Eddy's writings."

Each "Scientist" is supposed to treat himself, but should the erroneous belief in the sickness of his body not yield to his efforts, a Christian Science healer or practitioner may be called in. The proper prelude to the ministrations of the healer must be that he, himself, comes with the right attitude. For him, sickness is a dream from which the person needs to be awakened.[2] In the words of a

---

[1] Kimball, E. A.: *Answers to Questions Concerning Christian Science.* Boston, The Christian Science Publishing Society, 1909.

[2] Eddy, M. B.: *Science and Health.* Boston, Christian Science Publishing Society, 1934.

Christian Scientist, the practitioner "denies the claims of mortal mind and awakens the thought of the patient to the fact that God, Divine Mind, did not make sickness, and therefore sickness is an illusion which will disappear upon his maintaining the true facts about man's being." He treats each symptom of the disease in turn, refutes the testimony of the material senses and repeatedly affirms the health of the patient. He will quote or read suitable passages from Mrs. Eddy's writings; there will be prayers. A treatment may last from a few moments to several hours.

It is not always necessary for the religious practitioner to treat in person. He may give absent treatment, the assumption being that one mind is able to have an effect upon another even at a distance, and that the prayers and affirmations of the practitioner will be hardly less effective in absentia than in the patient's presence.

This method of healing is applicable to all disease—organic or functional, serious or trivial—necessarily so, because a belief in cancer has no better basis than a belief in a stomach ache. Both are equally erroneous. The Christian Science healer makes no diagnosis. Indeed, Mrs. Eddy remarks, "A physical diagnosis of disease —since mortal mind must be the cause of disease—tends to induce disease."

Role of the Physician   The Christian Scientist departs entirely from the modes and bases of medical science in his approach to disease and in his practice. To Christian Scientists, medical science and practice generally are only a tremendous fabric of make-believe. Whatever success doctors may obtain derives from the patient's faith in them and their remedies, Mrs. Eddy believed. ". . . Faith in the drug is the sole factor in the cure," she wrote. Christian Scientists, if they are true to the teachings of the founder, will not turn to medical practitioners and their measures, except in certain special situations. As a general rule, Christian Science practitioners will not treat a case unless the patient has chosen between his ministrations and those of a medical physician.

Under what circumstances then does the "Scientist" employ

the services of a physician or dentist?[1] First, they almost universally have doctors present during childbirth. "The physical conditions incident to the birth need a well-practiced hand." "The actual attendance upon the birth process would be considered a legitimate exception to the absolute requirements of Christian Science." However, the medical program of supervision during pregnancy is abhorred and a "deep study of the Bible and Mrs. Eddy's writings" is advised at that time.

Secondly, a doctor may be obtained in the case of a fracture. Mrs. Eddy stated explicitly, "Until the advancing age admits the efficacy and supremacy of Mind, *it is better for Christian Scientists to leave surgery and the adjustment of broken bones and dislocations to the fingers of a surgeon,* while the mental healer confines himself chiefly to mental reconstruction and to the prevention of inflammation. Christian Science is always the most skillful surgeon, but surgery is the branch of its healing which will be last acknowledged." In referring to "surgery," Mrs. Eddy evidently means the surgery of trauma.

Thirdly, Christian Scientists may go to dentists as frequently or as infrequently as do other people for the cleaning and filling of teeth, but the dentists are not permitted the treatment of a diseased condition of the mouth or gums. Finally, "Scientists" generally prefer, for obvious reasons, to obtain reading glasses from optometrists rather than ophthalmologists.

Mrs. Eddy provided in *Science and Health* that the question of seeking the aid of a doctor is up to the individual and that "the church does not control the individual members in the sense of dominating their thinking and decisions."

Mind Cure   Psychiatry, of course, has no part in Christian Science, but as one might expect from such a positive psychological system the psychosomatic ailments are rare amongst these people. However, the death rate from organic disease is much higher as demonstrated by Dr. Gale E. Wilson,[2] autopsy surgeon

---

[1] Hoffman, L.: Problem Patient: The Christian Scientist. *Medical Economics,* pp. 265-283 (Dec.) 1956.

[2] Wilson, G. E.: Christian Science and Longevity. *J. Forensic Science,* 1:43-60 (Oct.) 1956.

in King County, Washington. During the period 1935-55, he noted 1,041 deaths of known Christian Scientists. His analysis of those deaths provides the following statistics:

Average age at death was about 70—slightly below the latest figure for the state's population as a whole.

In twenty-one years, there were only three deaths from trauma, none at all from homicide or suicide.

The proportion of deaths from coronary artery disease was far below the national average.

The proportion of deaths from pneumonia, diabetes, and tuberculosis was higher than average.

The proportion of deaths from malignancy was nearly double the national average. But the incidence of carcinoma of the lung was very low. (Christian Scientists do not as a rule use tobacco or alcohol.)

Dr. Wilson estimates that six per cent of "Scientist" deaths could be prevented by surgery which is condoned by the church, although many do not realize it.

Supplementary Reading

Beazley, N.: *The Cross and the Crown*. Boston, Little Brown Company, 1952.

Bellwald, A. M.: *Christian Science and the Catholic Faith, Including a Brief Account of New Thought and Other Modern Mental Healing Movements*. New York, The Macmillan Company, 1922.

Dawson, G. G.: *Healing: Pagan and Christian*. London, Society for Promoting Christian Knowledge, 1935.

Doorly, J. W.: *Talks on Christian Science Practice*. New York, E. Becker, 1950.

Flower, B. O.: *Christian Science as a Religious Belief and a Therapeutic Agent*. Boston, Twentieth Century Company, 1910.

Hall, M. P.: *Healing: The Divine Art*. Los Angeles, Philosophical Research Society, 1950.

Hastings, J., ed.: *Encyclopaedia of Religion and Ethics*. New York, Charles Scribner's Sons, 1911.

Paulsen, A. E.: Religious Healing. *Journal of the American Medical Association,* May 15, 22, 29, 1926, pp. 1519-1524, 1617-1623, and 1692-1697.

Rae, J. B.: *Spiritual Healing and Medical Science.* London, Society for Promoting Religious Knowledge, 1933.

Ross, P. V.: *Leaves of Healing.* Cynthiana, Kentucky, Hobson Book Press, 1946.

Orcutt, W. D.: *Mary Baker Eddy and Her Books.* Boston, The Christian Science Publishing Society, 1950.

Wilbur, S.: *The Life of Mary Baker Eddy.* Boston, The Christian Science Publishing Society, 1907.

UNITY

History   Unity School of Christianity had its beginnings when Mrs. Myrtle Fillmore was healed in 1886 as a result of her study of the "New Thought" philosophies of Dr. E. B. Weeks.[1] She had been an invalid for years and with this revelation "became whole" within two years. Her husband, Charles Fillmore, was slow in appreciating these ideas, but by 1889 he had accepted the philosophy and threw his energies into the publication of a magazine, *Modern Thought.* This man had been a successful real estate promoter and entered into this new project with the same zeal.

In its incipiency, the Fillmore magazine stated that "our views are not those of orthodox Christian Science . . . but we are partial to and endorse Christian Science." In fact, the name "Christian Science Thought" was used for a time, but in 1891 the title "Unity" was introduced by Charles Fillmore. "Silent Unity" is the inspiration of Myrtle Fillmore and represents a central institution of prayer in Lee's Summit, where a large number of workers carry on sessions of prayers for correspondents by mail and telephone.

The Unity School of Practical Christianity, as it is sometimes called, is basically Christian but not Protestant in the sense that it does not quarrel with other beliefs. The group known as "Divine Science" is of the same nature as Unity. One of its leaders was a former Unity member, Erwin Gregg.

Another religious body of similar belief is that called "Science of Mind" or "Religious Science," which is still headed by its

---

[1] Freeman, James D.: *The Household of Faith: The Story of Unity.* Lee's Summit, Missouri, Unity School of Christianity, 1951.

founder, Ernest Holmes. All three of these movements stress affirmative faith that goes beyond medical science, but they do believe in working with and "through" the physician with prayer.

Nature of Disease   Unity rejects the "original sin" concept. It accepts disease as real, but preventable by prayer and right thinking. It has maintained a disbelief in hereditary disease as a result of Myrtle Fillmore's experience. The evolution of this movement through the years has brought it into a middle ground between the radical rejection of medical science (with certain exceptions) of Christian Science and the closely cooperative position of Christian orthodoxy. Today, the Unity leaders work with physicians, believing that their spiritual methods are an important adjunct to medicine or surgery.

Diet   There are no dietary restrictions whatever in the teachings of Unity, although as a matter of interest Mr. Fillmore did not eat meat. Also, there is no open taboo of smoking or the use of alcohol.

Role of the Physician   One of the present-day writers for Unity is a physician, Dr. C. O. Southard.[1] In his book the use of Unity healing in conjunction with medical means is described. The emphasis is on treating the "three-fold being—the physical, the mental and the spiritual," part of this is done by the physician and part by the use of the teachings of Unity.

"We shall have more physicians learning Jesus' method of healing. Doctors of the future will not so often say, 'Put the patient in the hospital and operate.' They will say, 'Put the patient in the hospital and learn what's wrong with his thinking.' And when they find out, they can say 'Take up thy bed and walk.' For there will be great hospitals wherein people are taught how to think their way to health by learning spiritual laws and keeping them. That day is coming for all men and every good meta-physician who has seen faith or prayer healings taking place knows it is coming. And more doctors are trying to bring that day closer than some may realize."

Therapy   There is no dogma against birth control, artificial insemination, etc., in the Unity movement. It teaches that the mind has power to cause and cure illness, and that faith

---

[1] Southard, C. O.: *Truth Ideas of an M.D.* Lee's Summit, Unity School of Christianity, 1954.

eliminates both the physical appearance of disease and its mental cause. By eliminating such emotions as fear, anxiety, etc., many illnesses can be prevented and cured. "The solution begins in the honest facing of disease with the doctor, and with his aid ends in the development of a vital faith. A deep religious faith is the most effective cure, provided the doctor himself has such a vital faith to give."

Another writer[1] puts it this way,

"There are two ways to restore health: a long way and a short way. The long way round is to go to a competent and honest physician and have proper tests and examinations made. He will first seek the cause. In looking for the cause he will look into the body, mind, and spirit. He will consider diet, all kinds of personal habits. If still puzzled he may call in a surgeon, a psychologist, or a psychiatrist. For he knows the real cause may be hidden in any one of the three component parts of the patient."

"When treating for health in this shorter way, by prayer, you need not understand what is wrong as a physician or surgeon understands it. You need not know 'the subtlest unnamed relations of nature' nor why a cancer builds itself out of good blood and healthy cells into a horrible growth that consumes the host on which it feeds. You need know nothing of cell growth in order to be rid of ulcer, cancer, tumor, or any other growth or condition. You need only know how to commune with God, and to wait on the Lord and never once doubt while you are waiting."

Mind Cure   Unity rejects the idea that its results are simply due to suggestion or autosuggestion. They find no fault with psychiatry "as far as it goes," but it is felt that "psychiatry empties the mind, whereas Unity fills it with Faith."

Fillmore accepted the healing centers, such as Lourdes, but felt that this same result could be accomplished by the individual through Unity methods or through the prayers of Silent Unity.

Supplementary Reading

Beranger, C.: *Peace Begins at Home.* Lee's Summit, Missouri, Unity School, 1954.

---

[1] Mann, S. T.: *Change Your Life Through Prayer.* New York, Dodd, Mead, and Co., 1946.

————: *You Can Be Happy.* Los Angeles, De Vorse, 1950.

Fillmore, C.: *Atom-Smashing Power of the Mind.* Lee's Summit, Missouri, Unity School, 1949.

————: *Christian Healing: The Science of Being.* Kansas City, Missouri, Unity School of Christianity, 1928.

Gatlin, D.: *Prayer Changes Things.* Lee's Summit, Missouri, Unity School, 1951.

————: *God Is The Answer?* Lee's Summit, Missouri, Unity School, 1938.

Pomeroy, E.: *Powers of the Soul and How to Use Them.* New York, Island Press, 1948.

Whitney, F. B.: *Be of Good Courage.* Lee's Summit, Missouri, Unity School, 1953.

Wilson, E. C.: *Great Physician.* Lee's Summit, Missouri, Unity School, 1945.

————: *Sons of Heaven.* Los Angeles, Unity Classics, 1941.

INDEX

Date Due

1/11			
MAR 19 1974			
APR 2 1974			
NOV 5 1976			
FEB 2 0 1981			
APR 9 1983			
FEB 2 4 1986			
APR 4 1987			
APR 2 0 1989			
		PRINTED IN U. S. A.	